Bacterial Vaginosis

Identify your Bacterial Vaginosis symptoms and then try the different Bacterial Vaginosis treatment ideas so that you can find one that works for you and stop recurring infections

Ellen Vincent

First Printing, 2015

ISBN - 13:978-1502321749

ISBN - 10:1502321742

Printed in the United States of America

Dedication

For women everywhere

Bacterial Vaginosis

Table of Contents

Introduction

There are a lot of different chronic conditions that can affect the vaginal area of women. We are used to getting yeast infections that seem to come and go with a will of their own. We are also used to the visits to doctors and gynecologists where we are told that our great problem is just another yeast infection. It is no surprise therefore, that after a few of these experiences women don't even bother seeking further medical advice.

Rather than getting a diagnosis of the condition it seems less bother to resort to an easy fix by going to the nearest pharmacy or drugstore. There are plenty of creams or powders that can easily be obtained over the counter for such conditions 'found down there'. In addition to this they are also cheaper than resorting to a prescription medicine. As a result it certainly makes sense to try them out in the hope that they will do the trick and cure the condition. There are also plenty of family, home or folk cures for these conditions as well. This may include drinking juices such as those made from cranberries, having hot baths or even cold baths. With all of these quack cures it is no wonder that we become confused as to where to turn, or where to go for help.

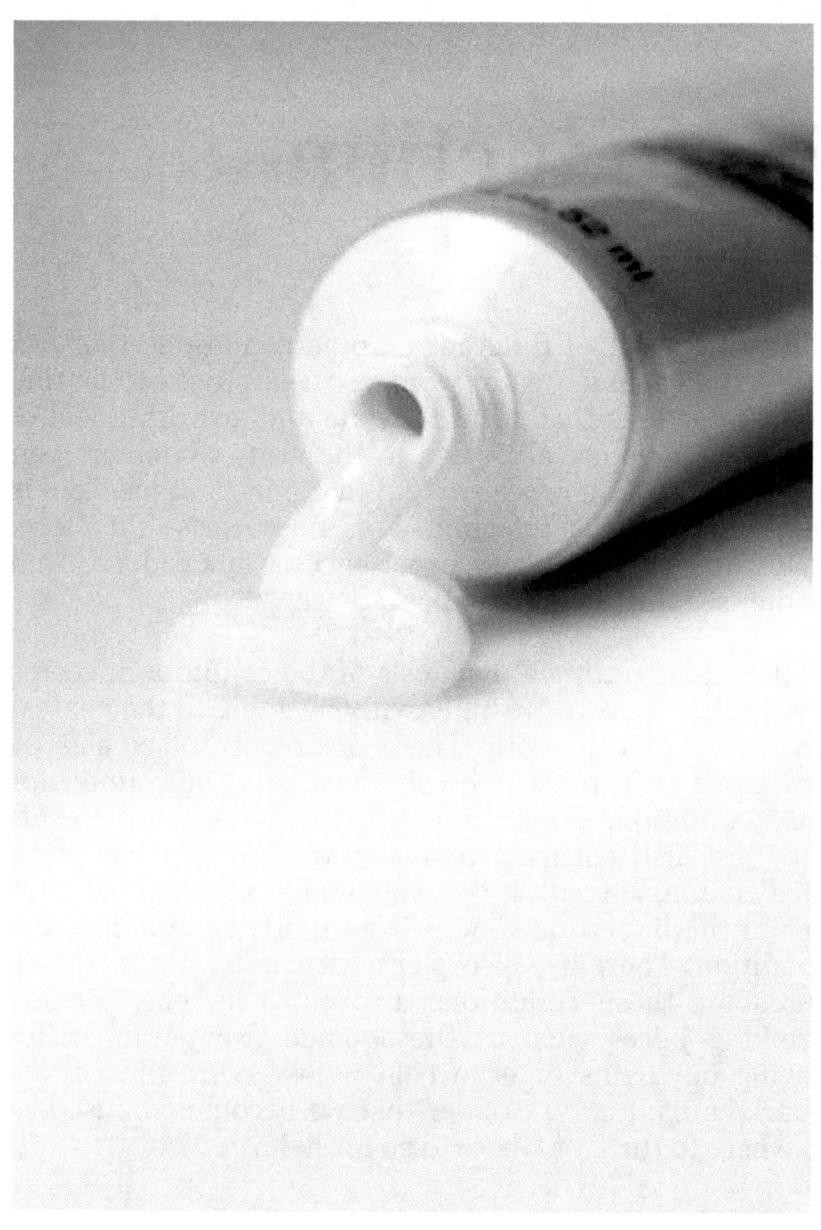

Instead of grabbing the first thing at hand, what we should do is to try and work out what is actually going on and why the condition keeps coming back. The sad fact is that, despite all of these treatments it is likely that we are actually trying to sort out the wrong problem. The continual yeast infection, that you think you have, may in actual fact be Bacterial Vaginosis. This condition is often simply called bacterial vaginosis. It is unfortunate that bacterial vaginosis may in a lot of ways be very similar to the yeast infections that we are used to. It is also often the case that in other medical conditions we may end up treating the wrong thing. An example of this is eczema and athlete's foot. You may have itchy toes and go onto think that you have athlete's and go onto use a fungicide to treat it. The itchiness goes away and you think you have cured it only for it to return again in a few days. This can get very frustrating unless you suddenly identify that the thing is eczema rather than a fungal infection. Here you can see that by making an assumption we end up using the wrong treatment. If only you had known that it was eczema you would have used the right treatment. Bacterial vaginosis is rather like this. There are millions of women who are busy thinking that they have a yeast problem instead of bacterial vaginosis and are hard at work treating it with the wrong things and then wondering why it doesn't go away and keeps coming back. In this way bacterial vaginosis can be both emotionally and physically exhausting. It can make people feel embarrassed and make them limit their normal daily life to fit in with it.

How do You Get Bacterial Vaginosis?

There are lots of myths about how women end up with bacterial vaginosis. A lot of these are similar to the ones associated with sexually transmitted diseases. Here are some of those myths:

A toilet seat used by an infected person
Sitting in wet sand at the beach
Lingering in public or private swimming pools
In a hot tub or sauna
Touching objects used by an infected person
Sleeping on bedding not properly sanitized
Wearing a wet swim suit too long
Failure to dry completely after shower or swimming
Wearing undergarments washed in harsh detergents
Lingering too long in a hot bubble bath
Excess use of perfumed lotions in the vaginal area
Sharing clothing with other women

These are not methods of transmission for this particular condition. However, a number of them can aggravate the condition once you have got it.

Bacterial Vaginosis is usually passed on during sexual contact. This can be between male and female or two females. Medical research has not identified all of the details about the transmission of bacterial vaginosis. Despite this it appears that women who have never been sexually active before rarely get bacterial vaginosis. This is not to say that women who have never had sex can't get bacterial vaginosis. There just seem to be a lot less of them.

Bacterial vaginosis is often misdiagnosed or not diagnosed at all by doctors and as a result it is difficult to get an accurate number on exactly how many women actually have bacterial vaginosis. From information provided by the Center for Disease Control and Prevention, it seems that about 1 in every 424 women is reported to have bacterial vaginosis. In terms of ethnic breakdown it appears to be more abundant among African Americans (23%) and Hispanics (16%). Fewer incidents of bacterial vaginosis are reported in Caucasians (9%) and Asians (6%). There doesn't appear to be any specific reason for these differences.

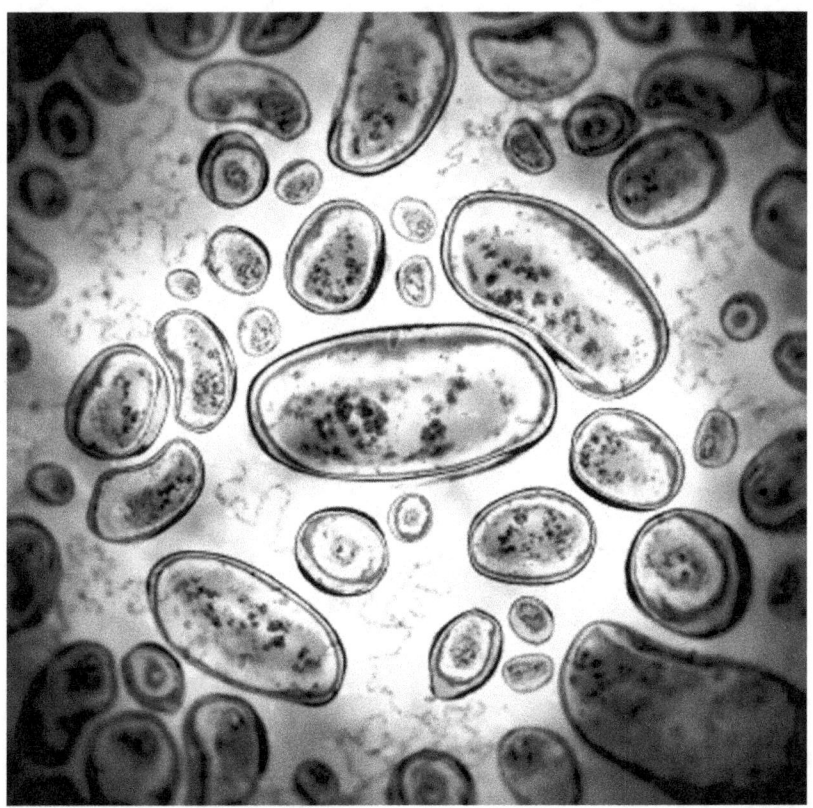

A healthy vagina actually does have a population of bacteria. These bacteria are the good ones. They help to keep away any harmful bacteria and maintain healthy conditions in there. A healthy vagina has an environment in which the good bacteria are more prominent than the harmful bacteria. A woman's body is constantly monitoring and regulating good bacteria in various areas so the balance tips towards health. Often, conditions outside the body lead to an imbalance, which results in bacterial vaginosis or other vaginal infections that require treatment to restore the healthy balance.

Bacterial vaginosis and Sexually Transmitted Diseases

Bacterial Vaginosis is not a sexually transmitted disease (STD). However, there is a lot of disagreement about its relationship to sexually transmitted diseases. In some medical areas it is associated with STDs because it only seems to affect those women that are sexually active. However, the fact that it only seems to affect women and not men is an indication that we shouldn't really call it an STD. The only real reason for talking about its classification is that STDs have a certain stigma attached to them. This in turn might cause some women to avoid getting treated for it. In its favor is the fact that you don't have to go to an STD clinic to get treated. You only have to consult your local doctor. The main thing to consider is that no matter how you view it there is no reason not to seek and get treatment for bacterial vaginosis. Don't suffer on your own just because the infection seems to be embarrassing.

Bacterial Vaginosis Symptoms

If you have bacterial vaginosis you will find that you get painful burning and itching in the genital region which can't be got rid of by using the majority of commercially available powders, creams or douches. In addition to this you will find that it won't matter how hard that you try to keep clean and fresh there will always be a horrible smell that you can't remove. People describe the smell as something like a fishy odor. It is also difficult to keep the symptoms to yourself especially if you are in a relationship. Having bacterial vaginosis can put a huge strain in any relationships that you have. Bacterial vaginosis has in fact destroyed a lot of relationships with the women feeling that they have to retreat into their own world where they can suffer in silence.

Natural bacteria occur in lots of places on the human body including the skin, nose and genital regions. Often the natural bacteria in these places help to protect the body against infection by more dangerous ones. There are good and bad bacteria. The conditions found in these places tend to promote the growth of these healthy bacteria. However, if the conditions are changed the bad bacteria can take hold and produce infections. Bacterial vaginosis is therefore caused by these bad bacteria taking over. A lot of treatments work by trying to restore the conditions in the vaginal area to being more natural and encourage the good bacteria to return. This in turn means that the bad bacteria will no longer be able to thrive.

Any woman is vulnerable to bacterial vaginosis infections. Although bacterial vaginosis has been linked to sexual activity it doesn't mean that this is the only reason for getting it. It has been found that even women who are not indulging in sexual activity can get bacterial vaginosis.

There are a number of symptoms that would indicate that you have bacterial vaginosis and these include

Thicker than normal vaginal discharge
Vaginal discharge that lasts longer than usual
Fishy or sour smelling vaginal discharge especially after sexual activity
Vaginal discharge that is white or greyish in color
A burning feeling when urinating
Feelings of itching or burning in the area of the vagina

This doesn't mean that you have to have all of these symptoms for you to have bacterial vaginosis. In fact some women report that they don't get any of these symptoms at all. It therefore varies from one person to another. However, having no symptoms may indicate that the condition has been established for a long time. This can cause long term problems as well as chronic discomfort. As a result if you suspect bacterial vaginosis you really need to do something about it.

Before making a definitive decision that you have bacterial vaginosis it is wise to consider that there are a number of other conditions that you can get that have similar symptoms. It is important to be sure that you don't have something else, because the treatments that you follow for bacterial vaginosis will more than likely not work with a different condition.

There are a number of different conditions which are rather similar to bacterial vaginosis and as a result it is important to make sure that you are actually dealing with it rather than one of these other infections. Bacterial vaginosis can easily be confused with candidiasis which is a yeast infection and Trichomoniasis which is a sexually transmitted disease caused by a parasite. Bacterial vaginosis is, of course, caused by microorganisms called bacteria. In order to identify the correct condition you need to look at the signs and symptoms given by each:

Candidiasis

This gives a white discharge, which some people refer to as being like cottage cheese. It causes an itching and burning sensation as well as pains which become apparent during urination and sexual activities. The areas infected may show a redness in color. Candidiasis can occur when people are feeling low or the immune system isn't up to full strength.

Trichomoniasis

This is a sexually transmitted disease and results in a typical fishy smell with a frothy yellowy greenish discharge. It can cause itching in the thigh area and swelling of the labia.

Bacterial Vaginosis

This results in a thin and whitish discharge which typically smells foul. This discharge is most commonly produced after sexual activity. Surprisingly there is very little pain or discomfort associated with the condition. Infection results in a change in vaginal pH so that it is above 4.5. Normal vaginal pH should be less than 4.5 which is slightly acidic.

The above descriptions can be used as an aid to self-diagnosis, but in order to be certain you should consult a health professional. Whichever condition you work it out to be you should also consult your doctor to make sure that it is treated correctly. You can also try any of the natural treatments described here in this book, but you should tell your doctor before using them to make sure that there aren't any other risks for you personally. People often try other treatments once they have found that medicines prescribed by their doctor haven't worked. You may need to try a number of different ones before you find a good one that suits your own body and personal circumstances.

Testing for Bacterial Vaginosis

Even though you think that you have the symptoms of bacterial vaginosis, as described in the last chapter, it is always best to get this confirmed by asking your doctor to do a test for it. There are a number of different tests that can be used:

A basic test used by doctors to make a diagnosis is to investigate the pH level of the vaginal fluids. This is a chemical measurement that determines the level of acid or alkali in these fluids. It is an important factor in knowing whether the conditions are right to allow the growth of the bacteria associated with vaginosis. As part of the pelvic examination, the doctor removes a small sample of fluid from the vagina to use for this test. This procedure is quick and painless.

Even a healthy woman has bacteria in the vaginal fluid. These usually cause no problems and are in fact helpful in maintaining a healthy vaginal environment. If Bacterial Vaginosis is present, the fluid sample will show an increase in certain microorganisms such as Gardnerella, Bacteriodes, Mycoplasma and Mobiluncus. Over time these harmful bacteria destroy the useful bacteria. A woman has no idea that this war between good bacteria and harmful bacteria is happening unless she experiences the obvious bacterial vaginosis symptoms as given in the last chapter. As irritating as the discharges associated with bacterial vaginosis are, it's an ideal early warning system that tells you when to get a checkup. The pH in a healthy vagina ranges from 3.8 to 4.5. However, when bacterial vaginosis is present, the pH level rises to about 4.5. This means that the fluids become more alkaline.

A fluid sample may also be viewed under a microscope. Here they will be looking for what are called 'clue cells' these cells will be surrounded by bacteria and indicate that vaginosis bacteria are present in the sample.

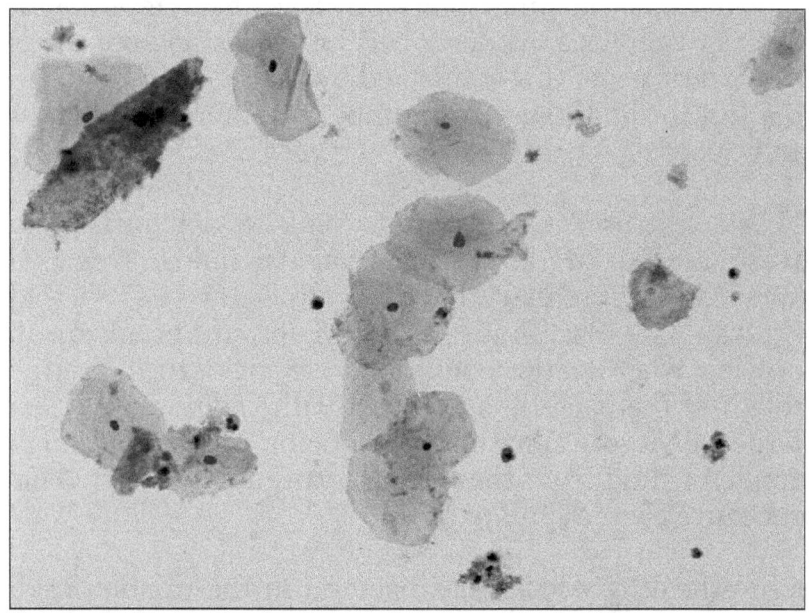

Gardnerella vaginalis bacteria on vaginal cells as seen under a microscope

A bold dye called Gram stain is added to the fluid sample on the microscope slide. Gram stain is used because it stains the various bacteria different colors. This allows the different types of bacteria in the sample to be identified. The gram-positive bacteria turn bright purple while the gram-negative bacteria will look a pale to pink color. Gardnerella vaginalis is a gram negative bacteria and is often found in fluid samples from women having bacterial vaginosis infections.

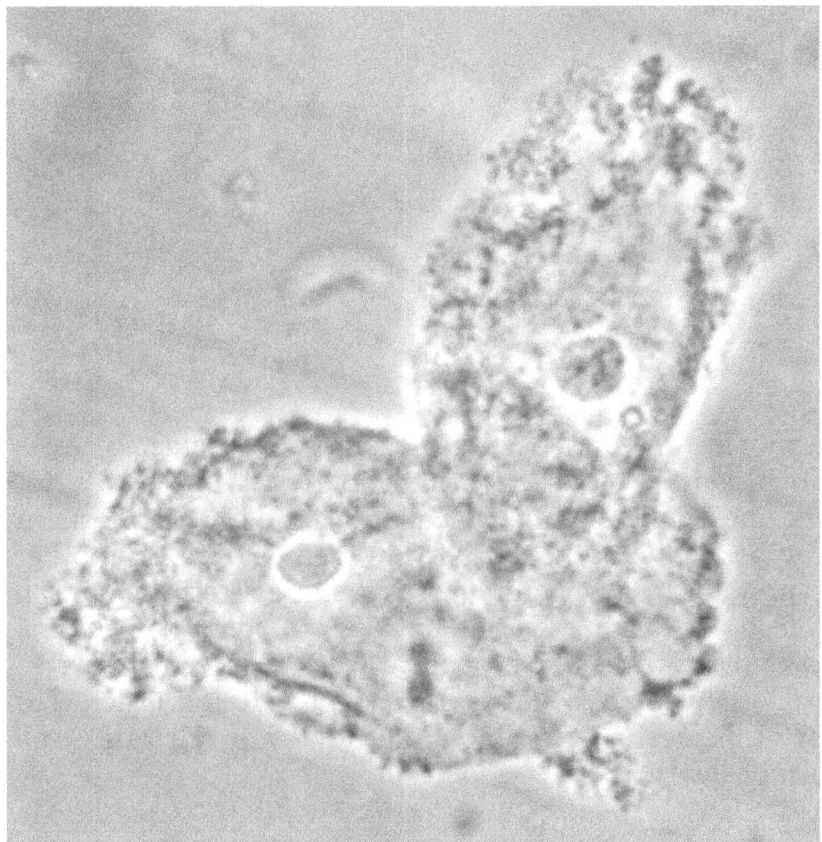

Clue cells surrounded by Vaginosis Bacteria

In addition to this, when vaginal fluid is exposed to the Gram test fluid, the typical strong fish odor is released. The test technician literally sniffs the test sample to identify that odor, which has become all too familiar to a woman who has bacterial vaginosis. Granted this does not sound like a pleasant job, but fortunately some people have the training to apply this process needed in making the diagnosis.

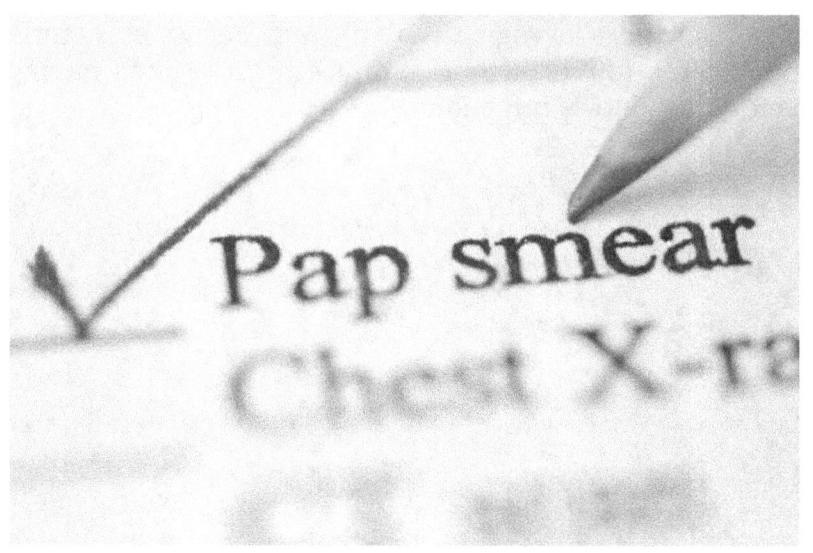

Another way that bacterial vaginosis is detected, by a doctor, is as part of a routine Pap Test. While this is not the most efficient way to identify bacterial vaginosis, it can be a help, particularly for women who show no other symptoms that would cause them concern about an infection. Relying on a Pap Test to identify bacterial vaginosis is not the best idea because its sensitivity to bacterial vaginosis is very low. As a result, if it is detected by this test, then the infection will already well established.

Because bacterial vaginosis symptoms are similar to those of Sexually Transmitted Diseases (STDs), the doctor may order additional tests for STDs. The strong smell that is associated with bacterial vaginosis is also found in two particularly dangerous STDs. These are Gonorrhea and Chlamydia. It is important to know whether the problem is bacterial vaginosis only, an STD or a combination of both. This will then allow your doctor to give advice on the best treatment option.

To get a valid test, women need to follow these precautions before having a medical test for bacterial vaginosis:

No sex for 24 hours prior to the test
No douching for 24 hours prior to the test
Eliminate all vaginal medicines for 3 days prior to the test,
regardless of whether the medicines are prescription or over-
the-counter treatments
Reduce acidic intake in foods and drink prior to the test
Reschedule the appointment if menstrual period starts

If you don't do this then any of the conditions given above could alter the results of the test. When that happens, you waste time going to the appointment and leave with a false sense of security. In a week or so, that feeling will be shattered as the bacterial vaginosis could return in an even more ferocious way than before, and you have to start the testing process over again.

Bacterial Vaginosis Treatment

When to get Treatment

You should go for treatment when you first see signs of an infection and not when you just can't stand it any longer. In fact there is no such thing as "too soon" for seeking help. It's also not wise to continue to tough it out in the hope that the infection will go away as suddenly as it appeared.

The most important first step is to get the proper medical testing to know the difference between bacterial vaginosis and yeast infection or other types of sexually transmitted diseases since many of them have similar initial symptoms. Many doctors don't wait for the test results to prescribe some level of treatment although these may simply be to try and control the symptoms initially.

This is not so suggest that doctors fail to take the problem seriously, but rather that it's a way to stimulate the body to repel the invading harmful bacteria. The idea is that the body's immune system can take care of things so the treatment is more inclined towards giving her something to focus on besides the bacterial vaginosis.

Other doctors are quick to prescribe general antibiotics, taking the "get in quickly approach" at the bacteria and hope to blast it away. The obvious concern with this is that bacterial vaginosis is prone to come back several times, and as antibiotics are the most common method of medical treatment. As a result this option can be used up far too quickly.

Over the Counter Medications

Over the counter medications are available. These medications are mostly anti-fungal, which can work for a yeast infection, but bacterial vaginosis is not the same problem. Women often resort to these because they are easy to obtain as you don't have to go to the doctor and get a prescription. In addition to this pharmacies and supermarkets which stock them are usually open at times that are more convenient. There are often ones that are open 24 hours a day. You may think that they would be cheap but once you have done some research you will soon find out that they are not.

Over the counter medications are not going to be as powerful as prescription antibiotics so you could spend more and suffer longer waiting for the cheaper treatment to work. The local pharmacy is a better option than buying from the supermarket or discount retailer as there is a pharmacist to ask for advice in choosing a product. Don't be misled by the advertisements touting the strength and effectiveness of over the counter creams or gels. The pharmacist will confirm, these over the counter medications are generalized and not targeted the way that prescription antibiotics are toward specific types of bacteria.

As there is no way to monitor the use of over the counter medications, the potency is not as high as that which can be given in a prescription medication from a doctor at the health clinic. On the other hand, an over the counter cream or gel may be better than nothing late on Saturday night when you simply can't stand the bacterial vaginosis symptoms another minute.

Any help is worthwhile, but you need to realize that over the counter medications only offer a temporary relief from symptoms because they lack the potential to cure a serious bacterial vaginosis outbreak.

Antibiotic Treatments

Antibiotics were the answer to a prayer when they were first discovered. This is because before this time there were no real drugs to deal with bacterial infections. Over the years as antibiotics have developed into more sophisticated and targeted treatment options, many diseases that formerly killed people were cured. As with any drug, there is the good side and the bad side.

Antibiotics are the Common Treatment for Bacterial Vaginosis

Antibiotics are intended to be heavy weapons in the war against bacteria. Antibiotics are not selective in the type of bacteria that they kill. They will therefore kill both good bacteria as well as any bad ones that cause infections. With Bacterial Vaginosis, the potential is high that antibiotics become "friendly fire," killing off more of the good bacteria than the bad bacteria.

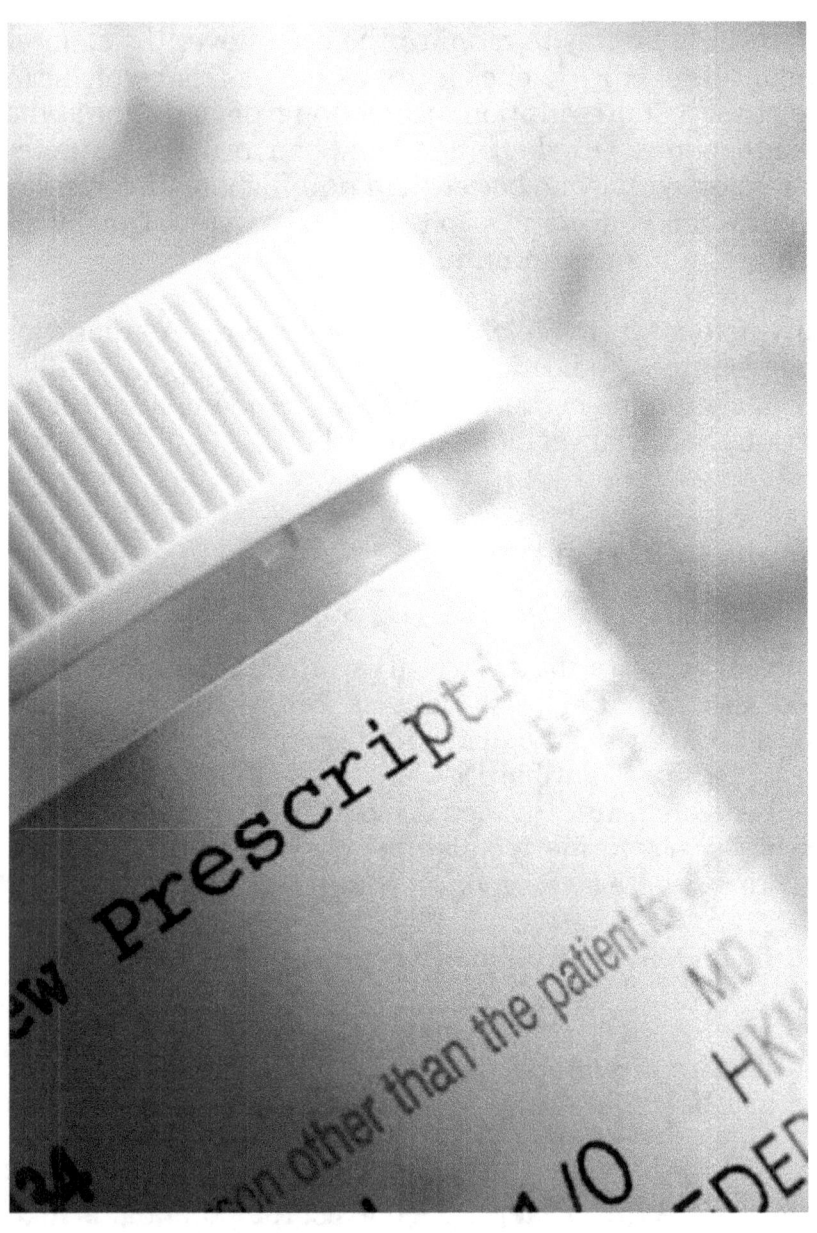

Generally speaking, the good bacteria are not as powerful as the bad bacteria so they are early causalities in the use of antibiotics. The good bacteria have no chance to repopulate the vaginal environment when harmful bacteria make the conditions hostile territory.

A major problem that frustrates doctors is that too many patients don't finish taking all the antibiotics in the prescription bottle. Even with the added instructions on the label plus the information sheet provided by the pharmacy, women don't read these important instructions. What tends to happen is that after a week, a woman feels better and notices less discharge or odor problems, so she pronounces herself "cured" and tosses away the drugs. While it may seem silly to continue taking medication after feeling better, it's absolutely necessary. The reason for this is that when you stop taking the antibiotics early there will be some bacteria that haven't been killed. The idea of using antibiotics is to kill all the bacteria off so that the good bacteria can repopulate the area. When antibiotics aren't allowed to finish the job the bacteria that are left will be those that are more resistant to the antibiotics in the first place. This allows the more resistant ones to multiply and this means that further prescriptions of antibiotics will have problems getting rid of them. As a result, if you are prescribed antibiotics make sure that you keep to the doses given and take them on a regular basis until they are all used up. Always read the instructions given with the antibiotics and follow them to the letter.

Oral or Vaginal Antibiotics

Prescription antibiotics can be supplied in either oral or vaginal medications. The question of better or worse is difficult to answer since what is better is the antibiotic that works fastest with the least negative side effects. Unfortunately, the only way to find this out is to use the medication.

The vaginal medications are in gel, cream or suppository form. While these can be messy, the advantage of vaginal medications is that there is less likelihood of experiencing the side effects, which can occur with oral medications. In addition to this the antibiotics are applied directly to where the bacterial infection is located.

Even though a woman may prefer to use the cream or gel prescription, those are not acceptable choices when pregnant or attempting to get pregnant. Vaginal medications are not considered safe for use by pregnant women because these medications are inserted directly into the vaginal canal.

Oral medications are easier to take and some antibiotics are only available in the pill form such as Flagyl, Tinidazole and Tindamax. Cleocin and Metronidazole can be prescribed in either oral or vaginal medication forms. The oral medications can be more precise in dealing with systemic infection; however they come with some unpleasant side effects such as:

Nausea
Vomiting
Diarrhea
Loss of appetite
Headache
External rash
Oral thrush (internal rash)
Metallic after-taste
Burning sensation similar to acid reflux
Vaginal yeast infection

This doesn't mean to say that everybody will suffer from such side effects. The majority of people will either have no side effects at all or will suffer only mild ones.
When taking some oral medications, the nausea and vomiting can become severe if any alcohol is consumed.

Even small amounts of alcohol such as in over-the-counter medications can prompt these reactions.

Some side effects signal a serious medical complication that needs immediate attention. The prescription information sheet provided by the pharmacy tells which side effects are the most severe.

If any diarrhea produced does not stop, the woman will be losing life preserving electrolytes that cannot continue to be depleted. Blood in the stool or severe cramps that are more intense than the menstrual cramping are reasons to seek medical treatment.

How Effective Is an Antibiotic Treatment for Bacterial Vaginosis

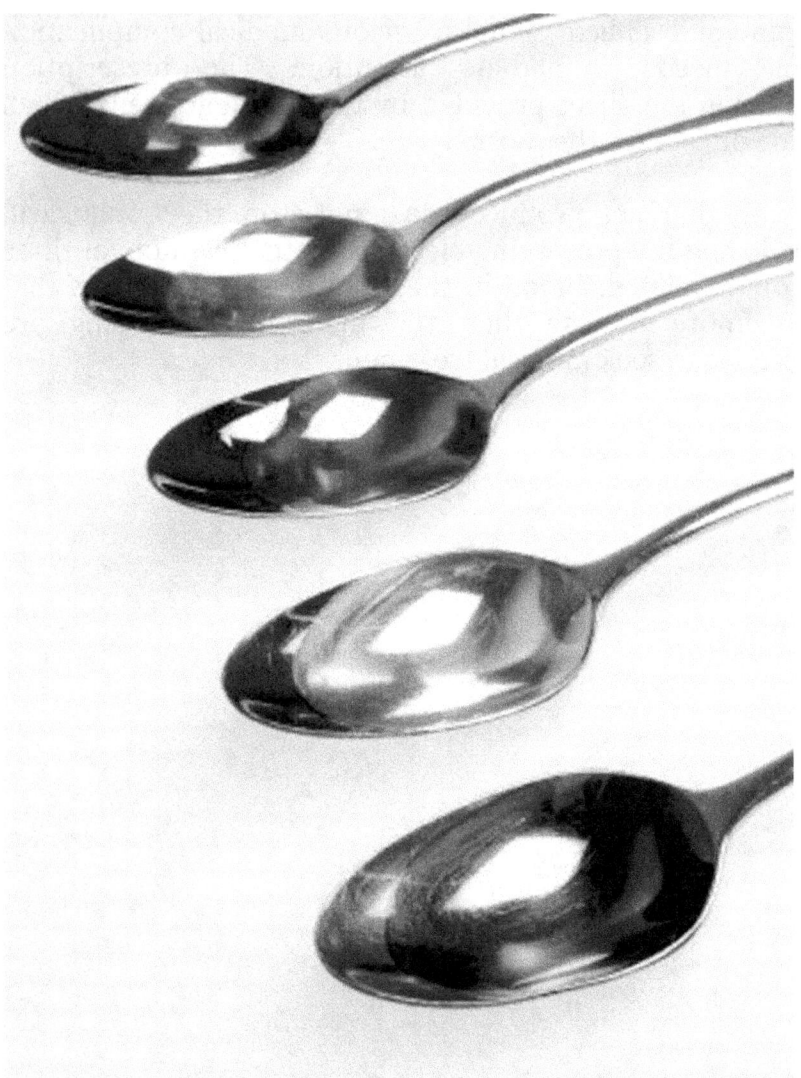

The disappointment is that after dealing with side effects from oral medications or messy vaginal creams and gels, the success rate from antibiotic treatments ranges from 50% to 90%. After all that effort and surviving the side effects you would hope for something more certain to take away the aggravation of living with bacterial vaginosis. The anticipation of getting help quickly for bacterial vaginosis is therefore not always met with the success level that is expected.

Failure to complete a course of antibiotics several times causes the bad bacteria to mutate, grow stronger and more immune to the same antibiotics the next time. Completing all the pills in the bottle, whether you think you need it or not, is therefore very important.

If the antibiotic that you are prescribed causes side effects, that are uncomfortable, you should contact the doctor and let him or her decide how to move onto another type of antibiotic.

The Downside of Antibiotics

All over the world people now consider that tablets and other medicines are the only things that will cure them. As a result we want to deal with any medical problem with a pill and preferably one that acts fast. Unfortunately, the same antibiotics that can eliminate bacterial vaginosis can also cause it to return again. This may sound strange, but it's a bacterial reality. Women who fail to complete all the antibiotics in the pill bottle or use all of the cream or gel are making it easier for bacterial vaginosis to return. Even if you are tired of bothering with the medication because you feel better, you shouldn't stop using the medication early.

The use of strong antibiotics or repeated use of these medicines can set up more problems than just those in the vaginal environment. Repeated use of antibiotics for any medical problem becomes a new problem in itself.

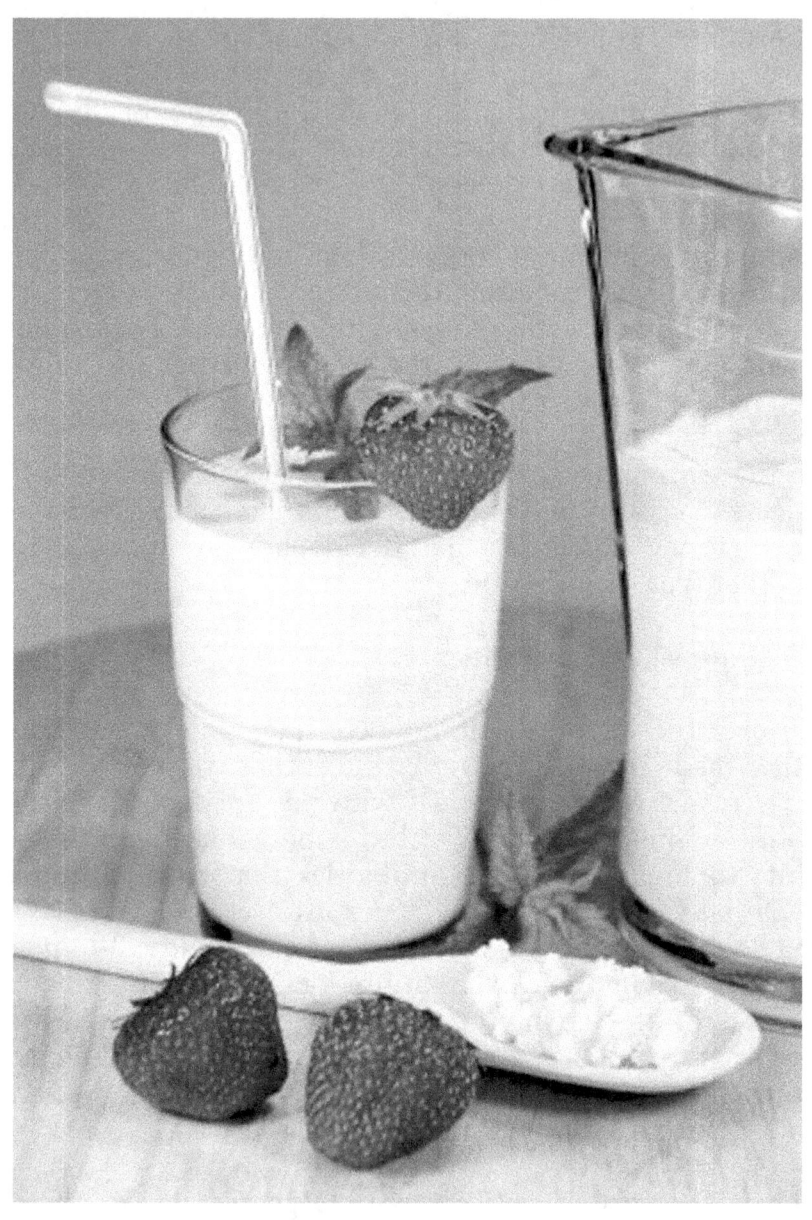

What doctors rarely tell a woman is how to deal with these problems. When taking antibiotics you should drink Lacto-bacillus milk or eat yogurt with Probiotics If you don't like milk or yogurt, probiotic supplements are available in capsule form from a health food store. The reason for doing this is that these drinks contain the healthy bacteria that the body relies on for its normal working. Taking these foods will help to repopulate the intestinal tract with new colonies of good bacteria.

Research has shown that frequent use of antibiotics for childhood ear infections leads to development of more ear problems. The same situation can occur for adults as well. When women take several courses of antibiotics, they are at a higher risk for earaches and sinusitis. Once that happens, they go to the general practice doctor who promptly prescribes more antibiotics and the cycle of symptoms will continue. Women must not be lulled into thinking that an antibiotic for bacterial vaginosis only impacts on the vaginal area. Once in the system, an antibiotic can affect any part of the body. This is particularly the case when oral antibiotic preparations are taken. Their effect is systemic as the blood transports them all round the body. The gels and creams have a more localized effect where they are applied in the vagina.

While taking oral antibiotics you can expect to have bad breath. That happens because the good bacteria in the intestinal tract have been reduced so much that the digestive process does not work efficiently. This bad breath is an early warning that the antibiotics have messed with the balance in the intestinal tract.

Even if there is no bad breath or grumbling stomach, always pay attention to replenishing the good bacteria that have been reduced by the antibiotics. This will help to avoid repeat infections of bacterial vaginosis or even a new yeast infection. It will also help your digestive system to function better and to avoid constipation from poorly processed foods that back up in the digestive system.

Bacteria Learn Fast

Bacteria are smart and they learn fast. Bacterial vaginosis has a remarkable ability to become resistant to antibiotics after the second or third time of treatment. For some women, that resistance can build up after just one course of treatment.

When the antibiotic medication is no longer effective in eliminating bacterial vaginosis, another antibiotic is substituted in its place. The problem is that these antibiotics are all chemically similar, and as a result it gets harder and harder to find one that works after several bacterial vaginosis treatments. This will also cause problems if you need an antibiotic to treat another condition such as a sore throat.

Not only are the antibiotics less able to fight against the bacterial vaginosis after several treatments, but some women find that the side effects are more dramatic and long lasting. It becomes a choice as to which is worse; constant nausea and headaches or bacterial vaginosis's smelly discharge and itching. Women in this situation don't know where to turn for help, particularly after taking medication faithfully and still having these horrible side effects.

Resistance to antibiotics follows a predictable pattern:

Doctor makes the bacterial vaginosis diagnosis and prescribes an antibiotic

Patient informs the doctor if she has any prior negative experiences with any antibiotics

Start taking prescription antibiotics for bacterial vaginosis

Within 4-7 days, patient feels relief from the antibiotic medication and gains a sense of hope that the bacterial vaginosis can be cured

Within the same 4-7 days, patient experiences side effects that are mild to severe
Patient reports side effects to doctor

If the side effects are severe, an alternative antibiotic is prescribed

The patient may have to go off the antibiotic early in order to get the severe side effects under management

Or the patient fails to report side effects to the doctor and as a result she decides to stop taking the drug

The toughest bacteria take the longest to eradicate so stopping or changing medications creates the conditions in which the bad bacteria thrive while the good bacteria have little chance to take back control of the vaginal environment. Each time this cycle is played out, the bad bacteria learn how to evade the antibiotic or basically ignore it. This sets up the conditions for a repeat of bacterial vaginosis, which is now stronger and more drug resistant than before.

Bacterial Vaginosis Alternative Treatments

It is common to resort to natural treatments such as the ones described here, if other treatments prescribed by a doctor fail to clear up the bacterial vaginosis. A number of women using such prescribed treatments as Flagyl or Metrogel find that it works at first and the symptoms disappear. However, after a short time, such as a week or so, it returns and the symptoms flare up once again. You should always try the medically prescribed treatments before resorting to other more natural cures. These natural alternative treatments can be considered as home remedies.

Women who have had one or more bacterial vaginosis infections know the frustration of seeking medical treatment, taking antibiotics and finding that for all their effort and expense they are not much better off than before the treatment. It is no wonder that alternative treatments are gaining in popularity.

Using Supplements

Those who know the irritation and embarrassment of repeated bacterial vaginosis   infections are looking for other options since taking more antibiotic comes with the danger of becoming drug resistant as well as developing yeast infection or urinary tract infections or both.

For these reasons a lot of women are not willing to accept whatever their doctors say. They are tired of having their complaints dismissed as not being a big deal. They want results and they want a say in the type of treatment to be used. At times that means women have to look at alternative medicine options, supplements and other lifestyle changes to control future recurrences of bacterial vaginosis.

Folic Acid

Because of the damage that antibiotics can do to the friendly bacteria in the intestinal tract, women need to be proactive in protecting their bodies. A simple way to offset this problem is to add Folic Acid supplements to their diet. Folic acid is found naturally in green and leafy vegetables. Unfortunately with so many processed foods and vitamin depleted foods, it can be a challenge to get enough folic acid in the typical Western diet.

The best foods to choose for increasing Folic Acid in the diet are these listed below. So be sure to add to the grocery list:

Fresh green leafy vegetables

Nuts, spouts and seeds
Whole grain bread
Bran
Liver
Lentils
Asparagus

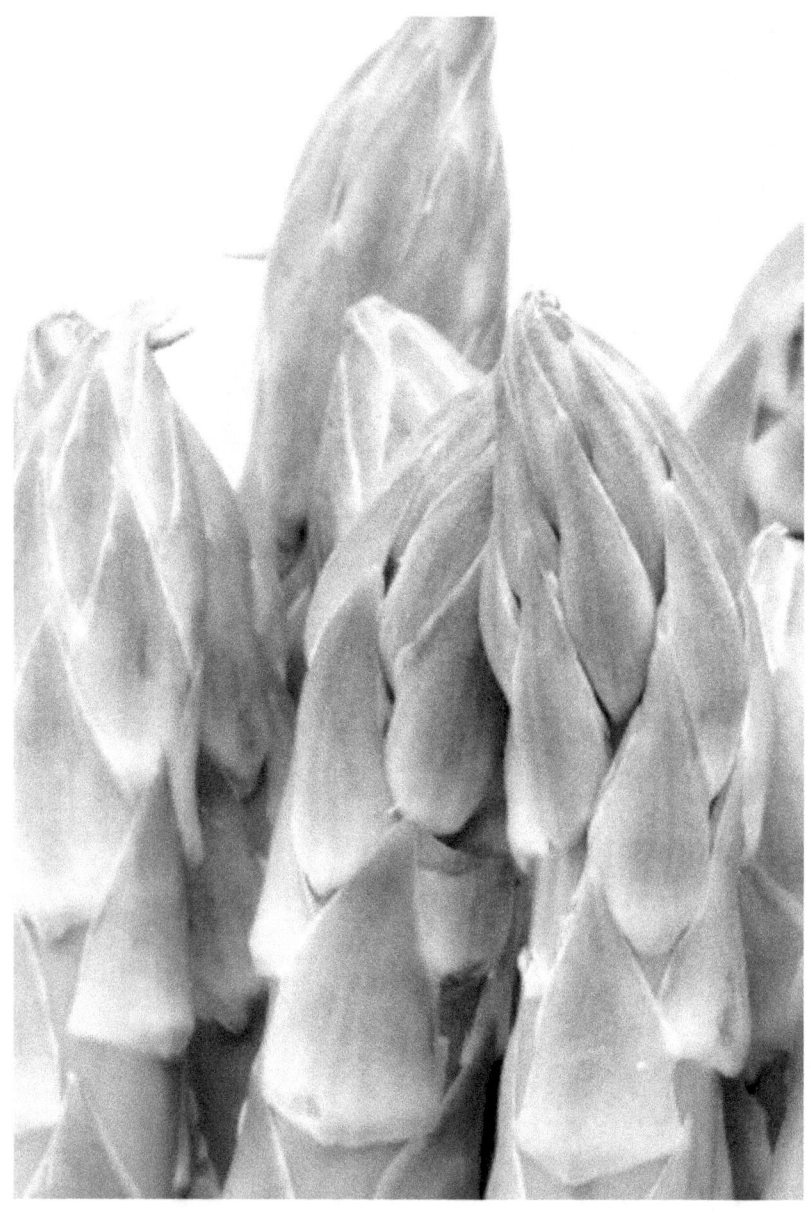

Citrus fruits like orange, tangerine and grapefruit

It is important that folic acid is included in a normal diet because the body cannot manufacture Folic Acid itself.

Although Folic acid occurs in many fresh foods such as green vegetables you can take supplements in the form of tablets or capsules.

The reason something as simple as eating foods with Folic acid can fight infection has to do with the way this natural substance works. Folic acid is a key component in producing healthy red blood cells and helping the body to metabolize proteins. According to the American Academy for Anti-Aging Medicine, Folic acid "increases the activity and production of antibodies and may reduce susceptibility to infection."

Folic acid is a type of vitamin B. Folic acid is important for the functioning of many chemical reactions within the body. Folic acid can help in the fight against bacterial vaginosis by strengthening the immune system and helping to restore the natural balance of the vaginal environment. This can help to exclude the bacterial vaginosis organisms as it doesn't like this balanced environment and doesn't thrive in it.

Folic acid is also known to benefit heart health by lowering the levels of homocysteine, which is a problematic amino acid. Higher levels of homocysteine are also associated with Parkinson's disease and osteoporosis.

Women with bacterial vaginosis are often not getting enough Folic acid either in a diet of fresh foods and whole grains or by supplements. The same infection fighting properties that Folic acid has for other diseases also applies to supporting the immune system in battling bacterial vaginosis infections.

The American Academy for Anti-Aging Medicine recommends 400 micrograms of Folic acid combined with a B-complex vitamin daily. Women who are attempting breastfeeding need to consume up to 500 micrograms of Folic Acid daily.

As with any supplement, pregnant and breastfeeding women need to discuss this with their doctor or specialist before adding any supplements to their daily routine.

Even with vitamins, more is not always better, so don't decide to take an excess of Folic Acid as a quick cure for bacterial vaginosis. The National Academy of Sciences warns that doubling the adult normal dose of 400mg to 800mg may be used for a short period with proper medical supervision. But in no case is it wise to go over 1,000 micrograms daily as this can create additional medical complications whilst giving no greater benefit.

It has been found that taking folic acid can work well with some women and it can certainly deal with any smells or discharges. Other women have found that it is best to combine folic acid with other treatments such as Acidophilus, apple cider vinegar or hydrogen peroxide.

Acidophilus

This is basically natural yoghurt. It contains acid loving milk bacteria which cause milk to change into yoghurt. These bacteria impart many health giving properties into the yoghurt that they make.

One of the best defenses against harmful bacterial infections like bacterial vaginosis is having enough good bacteria in your body. In the grocery store, you can find acidophilus milk, which is the best choice for people who have difficulty digesting regular pasteurized milk. The lactobacillus acidophilus bacteria are also in yogurt, which are often labeled "probiotics."

Women who do not like milk or yogurt can still get the benefits of probiotic dairy products by using acidophilus capsules found in health food stores. The best way to keep a steady level of good bacteria in the body is with the regular use of probiotics.

They can also be used in the treatment of bacterial vaginosis. The live milk bacteria release substances that can help to eliminate the bacterial vaginosis organism. One of the substances produced by Acidophilus is hydrogen peroxide. It also helps to reduce the pH of the vaginal environment to a more healthy level of less than 4.5.

Acidophilus can be used in the form of the yoghurt itself or in tablet form. In the case of tablets the higher the count of live acidophilus cells the better that they will work. The tablets can be taken by mouth and inserted into the vagina where they help to increase the numbers of healthy bacteria. When these healthy bacteria thrive in the vagina they can displace the bad bacterial vaginosis ones.

You should remember to keep your acidophilus pills in the refrigerator so that the live bacteria aren't destroyed. Acidophilus also comes in the form of capsules. Usually these capsules dissolve in the vagina after a small amount of time and the contents are released. Some women have had better success by opening the capsules and applying the contents directly into the vagina.

Attempting to over-load on probiotics as a fast fix for the early days of an infection is not likely to be successful and could cause problems. Some women choose to introduce acidophilus by inserting it directly into the vagina.

While stuffing yogurt up the vagina may seem disgusting to some women, it's probably no worse than dealing with the prescription vaginal creams or gels that you get from the doctor. Just make sure you clean up well or the sticky residue from the yogurt becomes as disgusting as the bacterial vaginosis discharge. Don't use flavored yoghurts because, although they may smell better, the combination of strawberry banana yogurt and bacterial vaginosis is not very appealing in the end.

Probiotics

Probiotics are basically the same as Acidophilus in that they consist of bacteria that feed on lactose sugar in milk and produce fermented products such as yoghurts. In a similar way these organisms may produce hydrogen peroxide and can be used to return the vaginal environment to a more normal pH. Indeed, probiotics may actually contain the acidophilus strain of bacteria as well. However, another strain of bacteria called Rhamnosus may also be present in probiotics. Rhamnosus has been found to work in a similar way to Acidophilus. As with Acidophilus, probiotics can be in pill form or as a natural yoghurt. They can be eaten and, or applied directly to the vaginal area. Not all probiotics are the same so if you are going to use these you may need to try out a number of them before you find a suitable one. There are also some probiotics that are designed to be used in the fight against bacterial vaginosis . One of these contains the bacteria Lactobacillus Sporogenes and again works in a similar way to Acidophilus. They can be obtained in tablet form and taken orally or inserted into the vagina. They are best used overnight. It is usual to use half to 1 whole tablet each night. The actual amounts used may depend on if you get any irritation from the contents of the tablets.

Ordinary plain yoghurt also contains probiotic bacteria and can be used in a similar way to the other probiotics described above. Plain yogurt with added sugar shouldn't be used. You should also make sure that you are using live yoghurt as treated yoghurts will not contain the helpful probiotic bacteria. This may be referred to as natural yoghurt. You can eat the plain yoghurt or apply it to the vagina by using a tampon applicator. The plain yoghurt will help to restore natural vaginal pH and healthier types of bacteria to the vaginal environment. If little success is achieved with plain yoghurt then you should try a more specific bacterial vaginosis probiotic.

Boric Acid

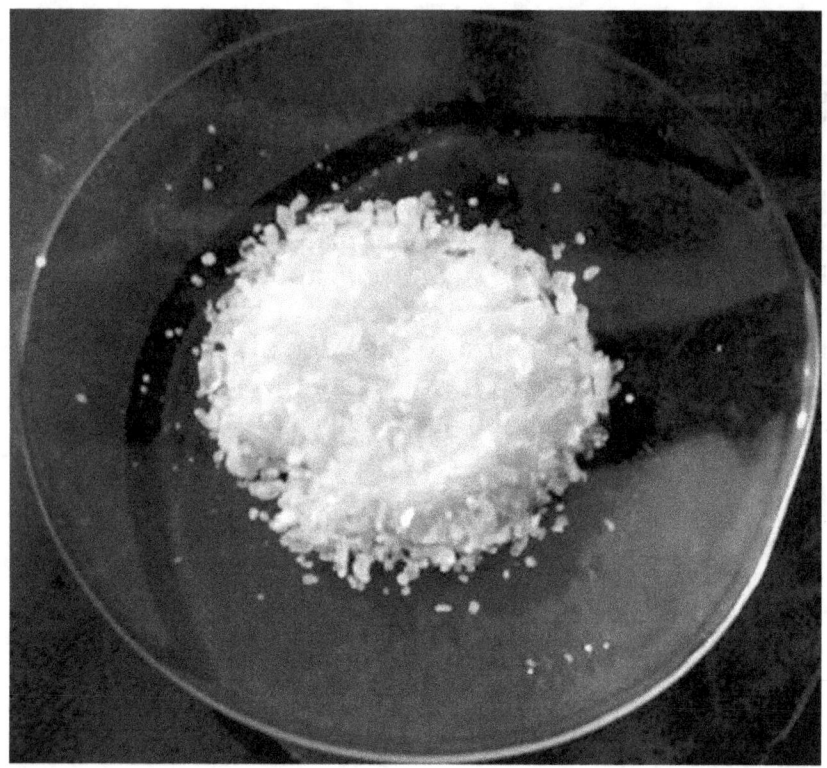

Boric acid is a slightly weak acid which can be used as an antiseptic. It is often used in the treatment of wounds and burns and may also be included in dressings for these conditions. Dilute Boric acid can be used in a vaginal douche to treat bacterial vaginosis. It works by helping to neutralize the alkaline conditions in the vagina favored by bacterial vaginosis and replacing it with a healthier acidic environment of less than pH 4.5. You can get boric acid in capsule form from the pharmacist. Inserting a capsule of boric acid into the vagina should stop any discharge or smell caused by bacterial vaginosis infections. Some people find that inserting one capsule of boric acid before bed on a weekly basis does the trick. Others have found that they need to use it nightly to start off with and also to use it after sex. After this you can take it once a week until the condition goes away.

Hydrogen Peroxide

Hydrogen peroxide has been used as a mild bleach and as an antiseptic for wounds in the past. It is a natural waste product produced by the cells of all types of organisms.

Hydrogen peroxide is sold dissolved in water as a 3% solution. When used as a treatment for bacterial vaginosis it is important to dilute it once again by adding equal amounts of distilled water. Distilled water is better than tap water because it is pure and contains no infection causing microbes. It is typically applied to the vagina in the form of a douche or on a tampon although other methods such as oral syringes may also be used. Whichever method you choose you should make sure that you don't insert it too far into the vagina. When using an oral syringe only insert it about 2 inches and make sure that you avoid the cervix. Proceed slowly and go gently. The aim is to flush the system out. Pressing the syringe or any douche too far can push the bacteria up towards the cervix and this is something you want to avoid. You may get a tingling or bubbling sensation during the treatment. If this gets too much you can flush it out with some of the distilled water. However, most women don't find the treatment too bothersome.

When it comes to treating bacterial vaginosis hydrogen peroxide should only be applied for a short amount of time which is typically somewhere between twenty and thirty minutes. After this time the douche or tampon should be removed. Some people get a positive result after the first treatment whereas others have found that keeping up the treatment daily for up to 5 days is needed to get relief. Although the odor goes away almost immediately after the treatment you may find that it takes up to 3 months before you are completely clear of the infection. It is important to only use the hydrogen peroxide treatment when you need it. This allows the body a chance to fight back against the infection on its own.

Some people find that sexual intercourse can aggravate the condition and as a result you can try giving sex a break or using condoms can help. It is thought that semen itself can change the conditions in the vagina such that it can encourage the bacterial vaginosis infection to re-establish itself. Sexual intercourse does seem to slow down the process of healing in this case.

Hydrogen Peroxide can be used on its own or in combination with other methods. Some people will swear by a particular combination of cures used together. One popular example is to use the following active ingredients and method:

Hydrogen peroxide, 400mg folic acid, Stress Vitamin B complex pills. Acidophilus pills

Start by taking 4 folic acid, 2 acidophilus pills and 1 vitamin B complex tablets. Soak a tampon in the diluted hydrogen peroxide and insert it into the vagina leaving it in place for about 10 minutes. After removing the tampon the odor and discharge should have gone. Continue to take the acidophilus, vitamin B and folic acid after the hydrogen peroxide treatment and this should keep the infection at bay.

Apple Cider Vinegar

As we have seen, one of the conditions needed for the growth of the vaginosis bacteria is that the pH of the vagina needs to be higher than normal. This favors the growth of the bad bacteria. Restoring the pH to a more normal, slightly acidic, level should restore the conditions where the good bacteria can thrive. This is where apple cider vinegar comes in. It is primarily a weak acid and should do the job that it is asked to do. It is also a natural product. No harsh chemicals here. Apple cider vinegar also has antibacterial properties that should see off the bad bacteria as well.

There are lots of reports that a number of women have had great success when douching using apple cider vinegar. This is especially the case where other standard treatments haven't worked at all.

You should remember that the apple cider vinegar needs to be diluted before using it. This doesn't mean that the original strong stuff is dangerous. It won't harm you, but it could be uncomfortable with stinging and some pain involved. Imagine getting vinegar into a recent cut. It would sting somewhat.

Here is a recipe that you could use to make an apple cider vinegar douche:

Add 3 tablespoons of raw apple cider vinegar to 2 liters of water. This is about 2 quarts. Use this mixture to douche twice a day using a standard douching kit that can be obtained from the local pharmacy. An alternative to douching is to use a tampon soaked in the mixture. It is best to get your apple cider vinegar from a health food shop as this is more likely to be the real raw stuff with all of the good stuff included in it. You can also buy apple cider vinegar from a fruit farm too. If you can get the sort that contains what is called the 'Apple cider vinegar mother' then you will have the completely natural stuff in it. Some people reckon that apple cider vinegar works nearly as well as hydrogen peroxide, when it comes to getting rid of bacterial vaginosis. To get even better results make sure that you take a probiotic supplement as a part of your diet.

Coconut oil

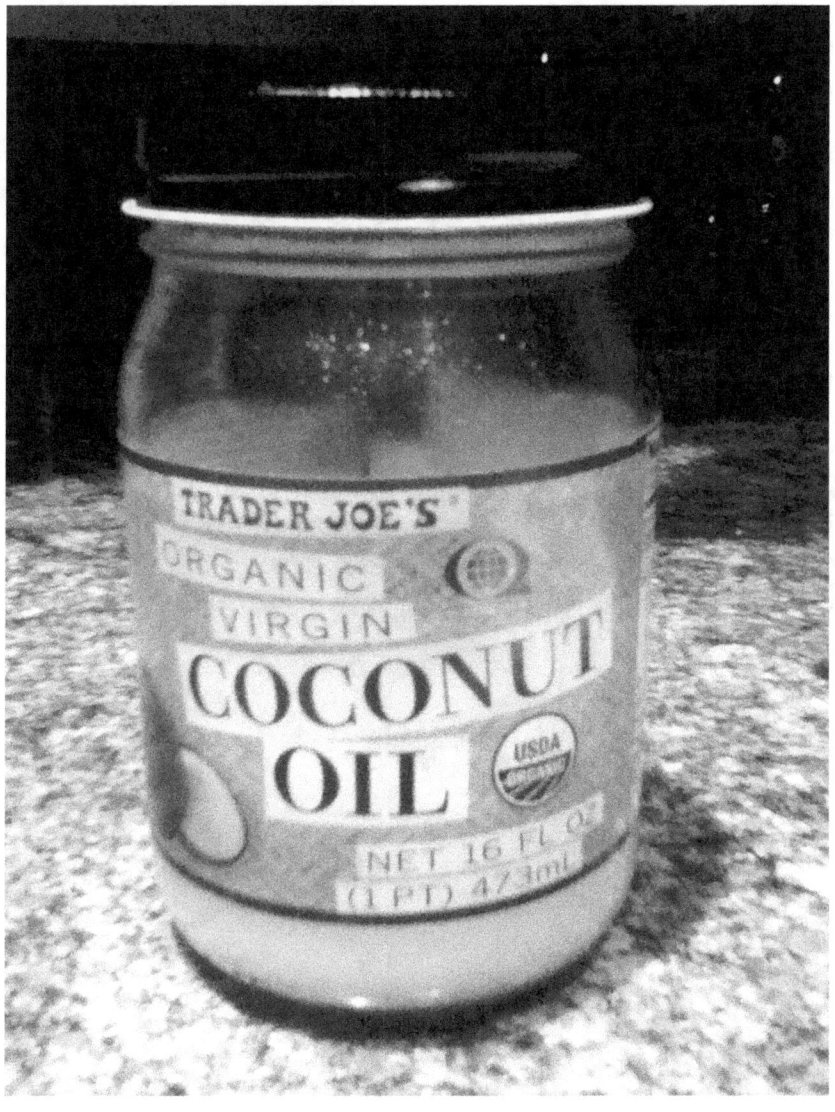

Coconut oil is a reliable natural product that can be used to treat bacterial vaginosis. It works because this oil made from coconuts has many other important natural substances included with the oil. It is all natural stuff provided by the coconut itself.

Coconut oil is fantastic because it not only kills bacteria but also kills viruses and fungi too. This means that it will also kill yeasts that are present as well.

You should make sure that you buy good organic coconut oil from a health food shop. Make sure that it is raw coconut oil and not a processed hydrogenated kind .

Using coconut oil involves a 2 pronged attack Firstly you should eat it with food and even on its own. When eating with food you can simply substitute the oil for any other oil that you are using in the preparation of the food. You can also eat it straight off the spoon or mixed with a drink such as tea or coffee. The second thing to do is to insert it into the vagina. To do this, first put it in the freezer for a couple of minutes. This will make it solid and then you can insert it more easily. Once in place it will quickly melt and do its job.

Garlic

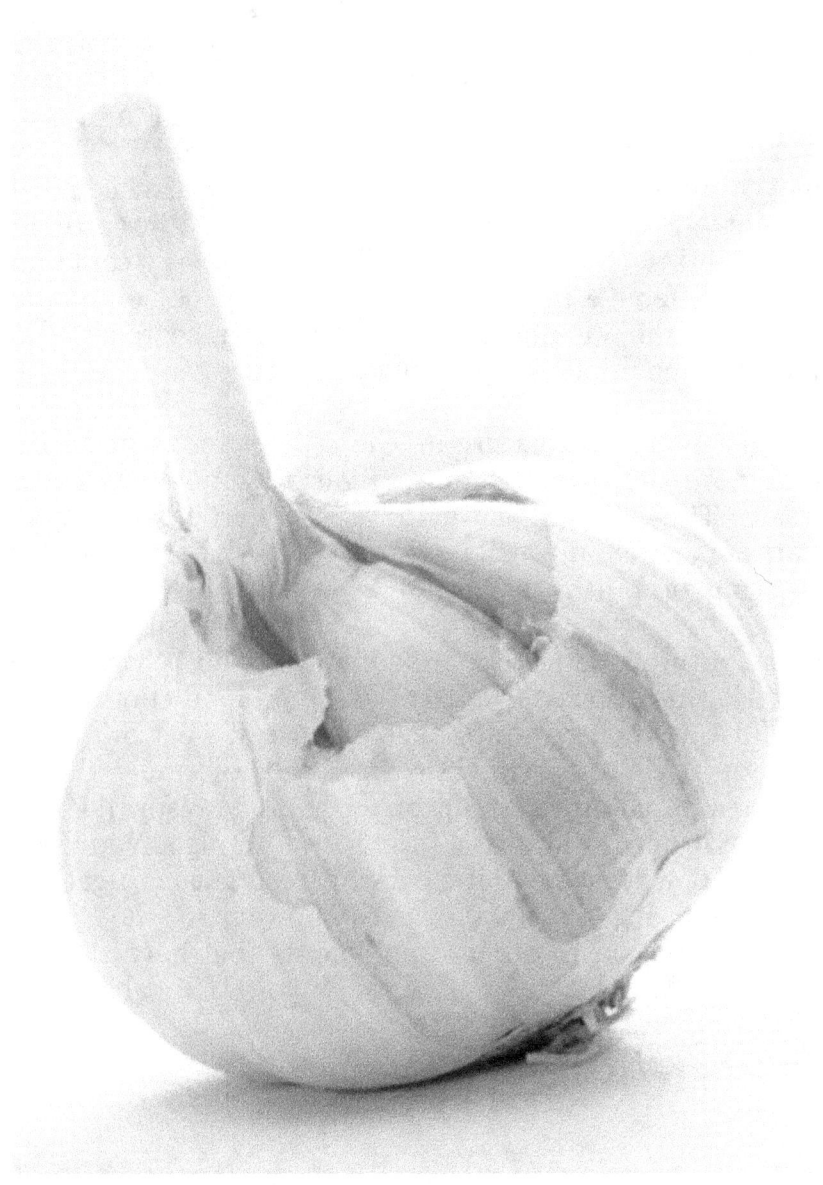

If yogurt is sweet and sticky, garlic is quite the opposite. Garlic is one of nature's antibiotics. In the late 19th century, Louis Pasteur experimented with a new idea discovered by a German chemist. This was that garlic contained a chemical compound that could reduce the growth of bacteria. This allyl compound, which gives garlic its distinctive and pungent odor, was found by Pasteur to actually stop the growth of bacteria. Nearly one hundred years later, a Swiss pharmaceutical company, Sandoz, attempted to use the allyl in garlic to create an infection-fighting drug. The company came up with an effective infection fighter but did not eliminate the odor so it was not marketed because researchers did not think the public would buy it.

The garlic tablets that are on the market today in health food stores have the benefits of garlic without the garlic breath. This is a kinder way to take in garlic daily rather than subject family, friends and co-workers to the eye watering, off putting odor.

Since garlic is effective in combating both viral and bacterial infections as well as lowering blood cholesterol, the little herb is a multipurpose cure. If you enjoy the taste of garlic, then you can choose to eat raw garlic or add freshly chopped garlic to foods. A few sprinkles of garlic powder on buttered bread isn't enough. You need to take in at least several cloves of fresh garlic to get the full benefit or a teaspoon of garlic powder. Garlic is best used in addition to other supplements that have a more specific effect on the bacteria involved in bacterial vaginosis.

Echinacea

Echinacea and Golden Seal are often promoted as natural remedies for reducing the impact of colds and flu virus. That's because Echinacea improves the immune system function by stimulating production of white blood cells that are necessary to fight infection.

One property of Echinacea that is particularly important for women who have bacterial vaginosis is that it is known for effectively treating both current and recurrent infections.

Another valuable property of Echinacea is that it can be formulated as an internal treatment or external ointment. The most efficient way to get Echinacea into the body and working on infection is to take it as a liquid extract. The liquid form is more rapidly absorbed into the blood stream than when taken in a capsule or tablet form.

In general, Echinacea is a safe, non-toxic herb to use. Since Echinacea boosts the immune system the only disadvantage is that this effect can become harmful for people who have autoimmune disorder.

Beta Carotene

This is a type of Vitamin A. Beta carotene is necessary for the production of the collagen that supports skin structure and cartilage for strong bones. Beta carotene is also an antioxidant.

High levels of beta carotene are associated with ovarian health, which is important for women who are attempting to get pregnant. When beta carotene is low, the ovaries are prone to infection, which can result in infertility. In the same way, beta carotene supports the overall immune system function and the maintenance of normal mucus in the vaginal environment.

Beta carotene is often combined with Vitamin E in capsule form that is found at the health food stores.

Vitamin C

Vitamin C is much more than a delicious glass of fresh orange juice; it is also important for immune system function. Like beta carotene, Vitamin C is necessary in the formation of collagen, which is the foundation for skin, ligaments and tendons.

The reason that collagen strength is important to bacterial vaginosis is that healthy skin is more resistant to bacteria than weak skin. Strong connective tissues are a secondary defense against infections that pass through the skin.

Stopping the spread of any infection gives the body's immune system time to launch a successful attack on the invading bacteria. Healthy skin is about more than looking good, it's also a measure of overall health and resistance to infection which is vital in eliminating the reoccurrence of bacterial vaginosis.

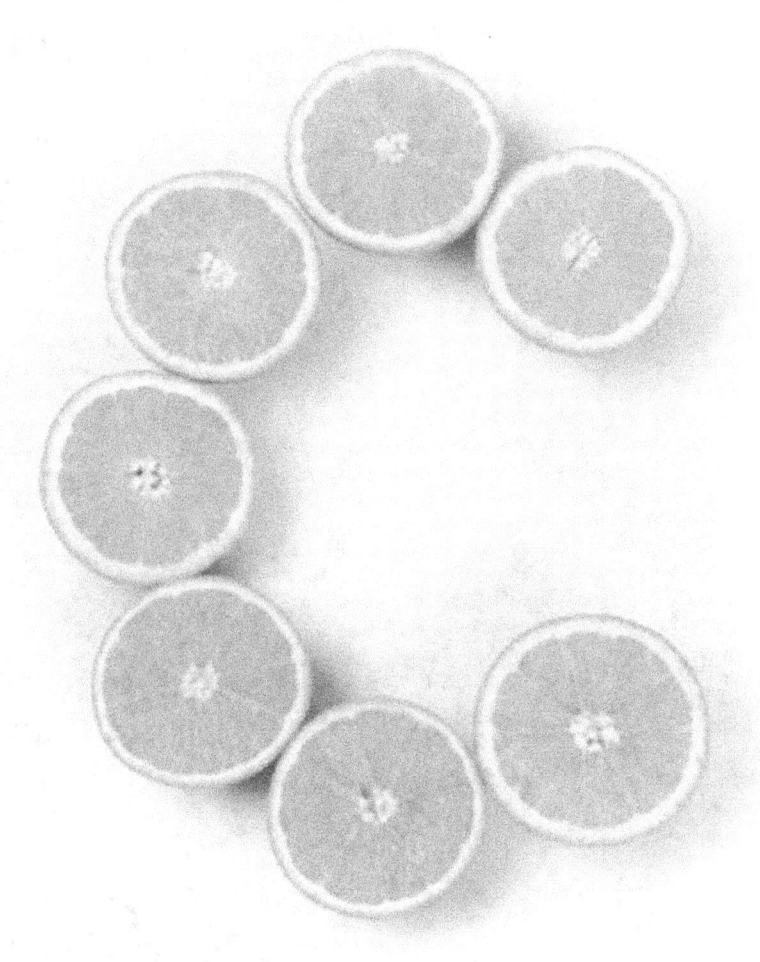

Myrrh

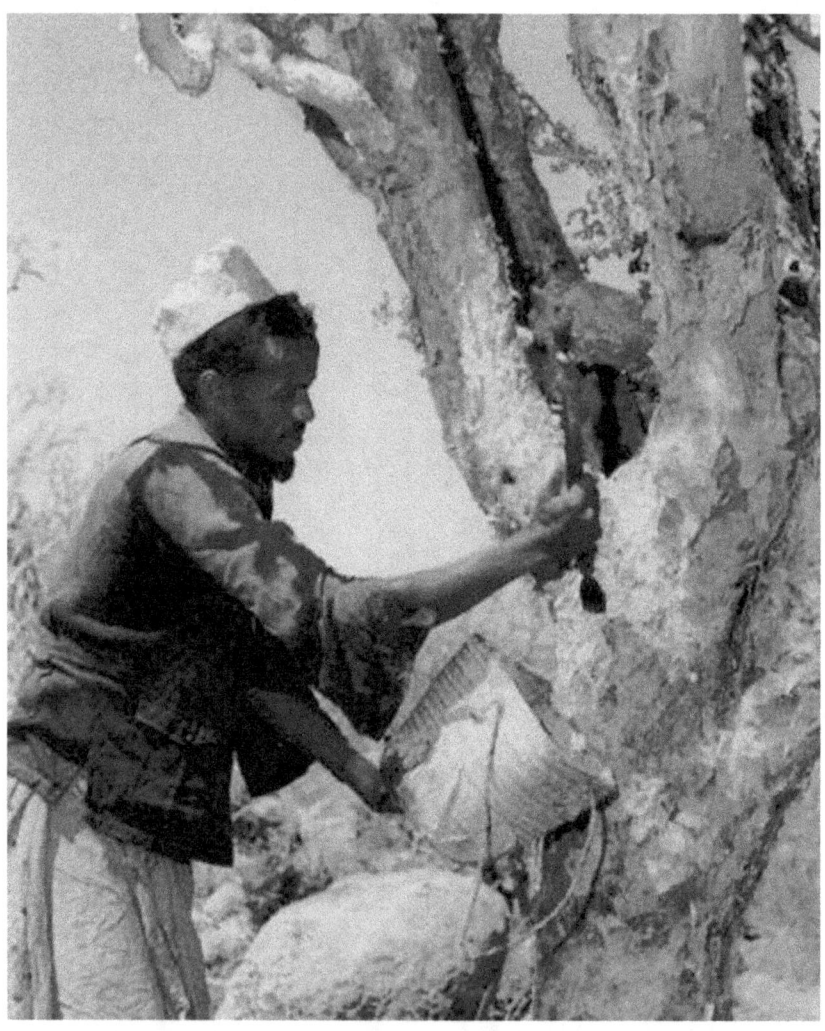

Yes, myrrh is something that most people only know about from the lyrics of a holiday carol. But in the Middle East and Africa, myrrh grows as a bush and is common among herbal remedies. The gum resin from myrrh is used in the Middle East for upset stomachs and respiratory infections.

Myrrh fights infections by stimulating the white blood cells whose job is to search and destroy bad bacteria. Taken as a liquid extract, myrrh can be used to treat sinusitis, sore throats, bronchitis and flu. In some herbal formulas, myrrh can be combined with Echinacea for extra power against bad bacteria.

Marigold

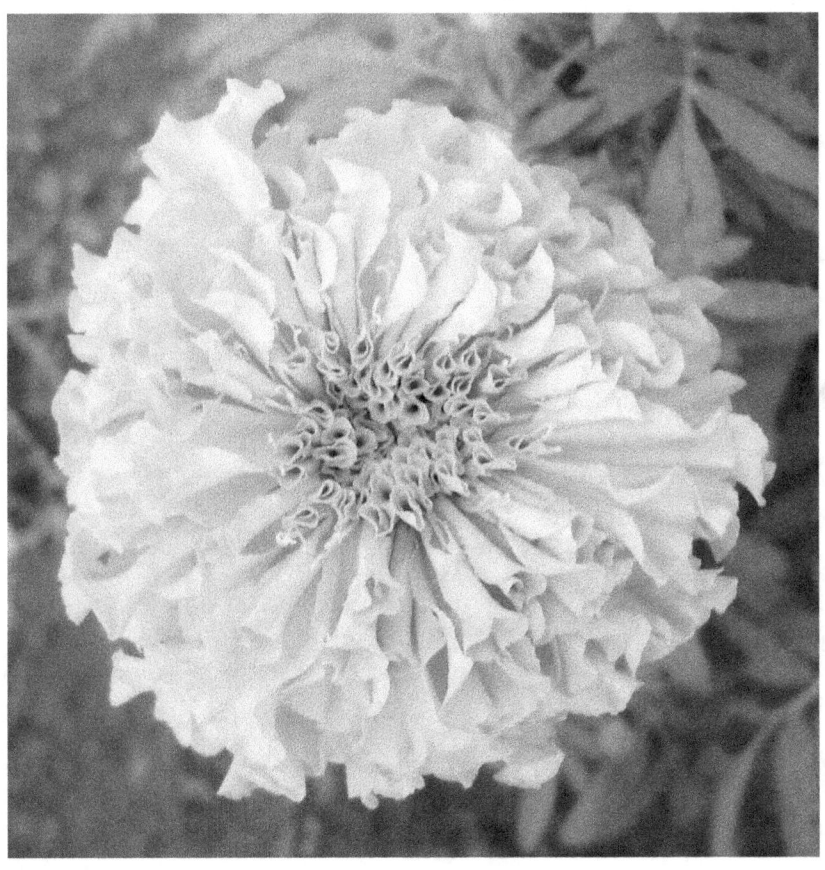

These beautiful bright yellow and orange flowers are as good for the body as they are pleasant to the eyes. Marigolds have been used for centuries to treat infections because of their natural anti-inflammatory and anti-fungal properties. You might be surprised to learn that marigold extract is found in many cosmetics, body creams and natural soaps. Marigold can be taken in the form of a tea or a liquid extract.

These flowers are so safe that you could pinch off several marigolds from the flower bush, place in a tea infuser and steep them in hot water. Then you can drink the marigold tea or use the marigold infused water to soak into a plain cloth and apply to the vaginal area for relief. You don't need to grow the flowers yourself as you can get fresh marigold teas at a natural foods store.

Tea Tree Oil

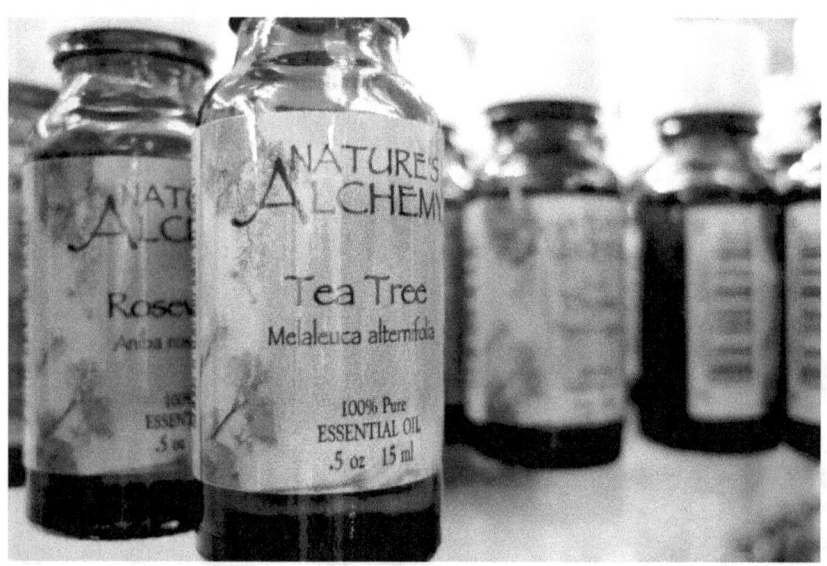

Tea Tree Oil comes from an Australian plant. In the outback, the leaves of the tea tree have been used for generations to treat burns and skin infections.

The healing property in tea tree oil is the terpeniod, which has both anti-fungal and anti-microbial characteristics. For this reason, tea tree oil is a popular element in ointments for Athlete's foot, toenail fungus, dandruff, eczema, lice and acne.

Tea tree oil has also been found effective in treating bacterial vaginosis and other vaginal infections. While tea tree oil is available in a liquid form, it must never be taken internally by mouth in that form. The tea tree oil extract that is found in toothpaste or mouthwash is sufficiently diluted to be safe for consumption.

As a treatment for bacterial vaginosis, tea tree oil is best used in an ointment applied directly to the vaginal area. Another option is tea tree oil suppositories that are made for vaginal insertion. Only use products made for internal insertion. Don't take external tea tree oil and insert it directly into the vagina.

Zinc

Zinc is a mineral that's commonly used in throat lozenges and over the counter medications to combat colds and flu. According to the National Institutes of Health Office of Dietary Supplements, there is a minimum daily requirement of zinc for all ages from infancy thru adulthood.

Zinc is important for cellular metabolism, wound healing and strong immune systems.

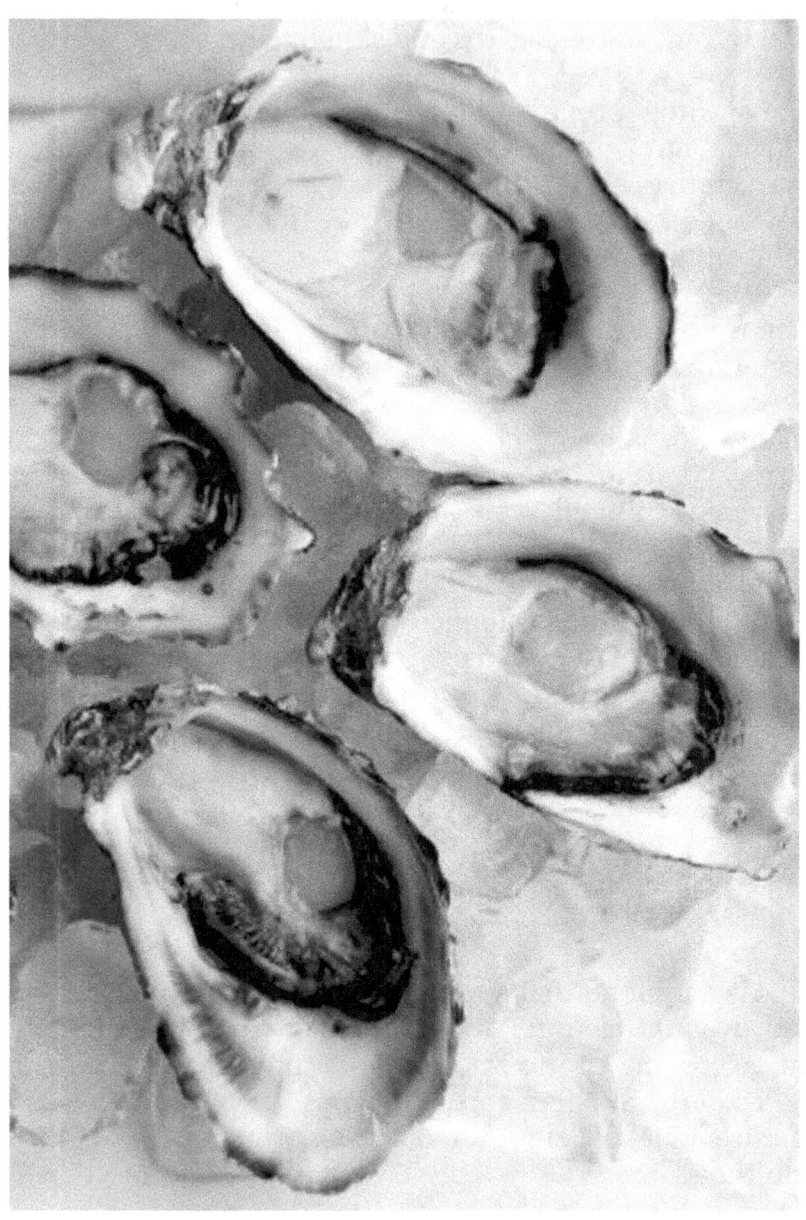

While zinc is found in many foods, oysters contain the highest milligrams per serving over any other food. Red meats, poultry, nuts, beans and dairy products provide lower amounts per serving but are the most common dietary intake of zinc.

When the body is low in zinc, the immune system is weakened. Without adequate amounts of zinc, the T lymphocyte white blood cells can't swing into action like the killer cells they are designed to be. People who have low zinc are also more prone to develop various types of infections and pneumonia.

With zinc, too much of a good thing becomes harmful. Be careful to take only the daily requirement for age and gender. The daily requirement of zinc also changes for women who are pregnant or breastfeeding.

One caution you should note is that zinc can interact with antibiotics, so don't continue taking zinc with prescription antibiotics without approval from the prescribing physician.
If zinc and certain antibiotics are in the digestive tract at the same time, they counter act each other so that both the zinc and the antibiotic become useless.

According to the U.S. Department of Agriculture Dietary Guidelines for Americans 2005, the best way to get regular zinc in the safest way is with a diet rich in:

Lean red meat
Poultry
Fish
Eggs
Nuts – cashews and almonds
Whole grains
Milk and dairy products
Zinc fortified cereal

Chickpeas
Fresh green leafy vegetables

Some multi-vitamins contain zinc so carefully evaluate the amount of zinc you get from daily vitamins before deciding how much additional zinc to take as part of the natural plan to manage bacterial vaginosis.

Green Tea

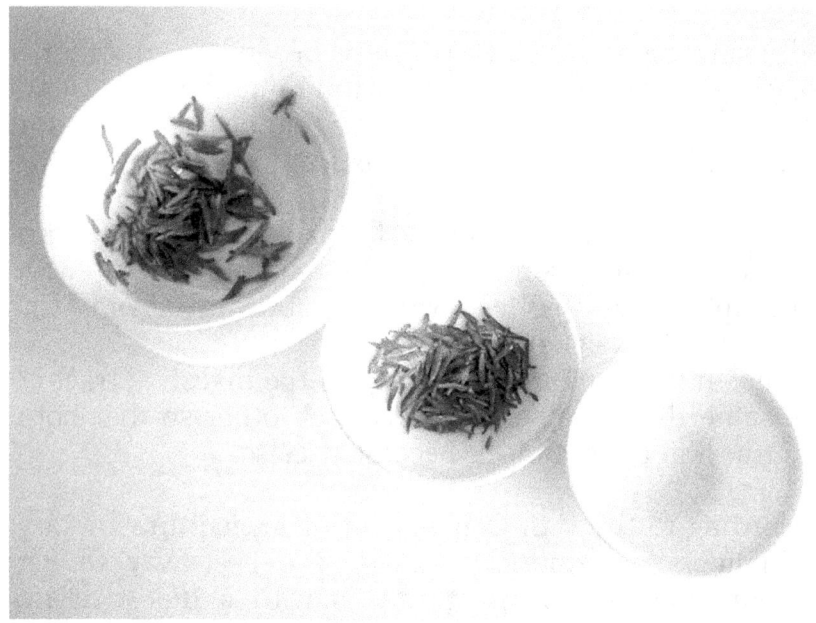

Even more than black tea or oolong tea, green tea is loaded with antioxidant properties. Green tea is a rarity in that it's something medicinal that also tastes delicious.

Widely researched as an immune system booster, green tea also delivers relief from irritable bowel syndrome, stomach upset, herpes simplex and helps to regular blood sugar for persons with diabetes. The anti-viral properties of green tea are also used as an element in an external cream or ointment applied to cuts, cold sores, acne and other skin infections.

Applying moist tea bags to the vaginal area might feel soothing but could be too much warmth and moisture. Instead look for an organic vaginal cream or gel that contains green tea or dap on concentrated green tea to the vulva, then dry off.

Green tea does contain caffeine so unless you get a decaf green tea, avoid drinking the tea before bedtime. If you are sensitive to caffeine or have anemia, you will want to drink green tea in moderation.

Aloe Vera

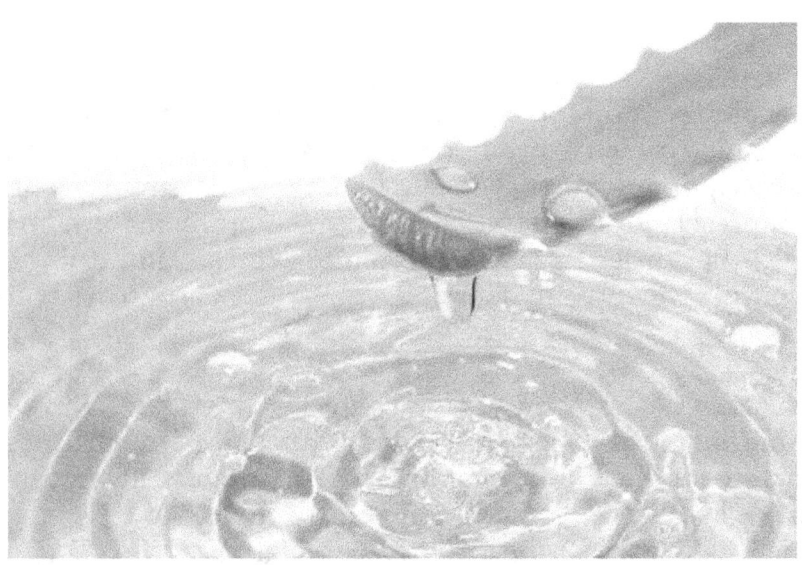

Inside this humble cactus is a powerful, natural gel substance with broad medicinal uses. When you break open a stem from this plant, you can squeeze out a clear gel that is a broadly effective for soothing irritants, itching and infections.

Commercially processed aloe vera is widely used in creams and ointments for burns, sunburns, cuts, scratches, rashes and insect bites. Some cooks keep a small aloe vera plant in the kitchen window as a natural treatment for quick access to treat a burn or scrape when preparing meals.

The aloe vera gel is also processed for use in internal remedies. Some vaginal creams or gels contain aloe vera, which can be applied to the vulva area for relief from the itching. The aloe vera not only provides comfort but also helps in fighting infection.

Treatment Conflicts

Whether you choose herbal treatment or prescription antibiotics, don't combine these without knowing the possible conflicts. The information sheet that comes with prescription drugs will list both prescription and nonprescription items that may cause problems if taken with that drug. Pay careful attention to this and call the pharmacist or your doctor if you aren't certain what it means.

The same warning goes for herbal treatments. Even innocent herbs when combined with prescription drugs can create the kind of chemical reaction that either boosts or destroys the prescription effect. In either case, the bacterial vaginosis is problem enough so don't add a prescription conflict to the mix.

What do Doctors Think?

Bacterial Vaginosis is often diagnosed wrongly as a yeast infection due to the symptoms being very similar. As doctors have to deal with so many yeast infection problems, it is easy for them to accept that this is the problem and not even consider doing a test for bacterial vaginosis.

Due to the link with sexual activity there are a number of doctors who simply blame unprotected sex or too much sex for the problem. They then advise women to go away and sort those issues out as their first line of treatment. Obviously this won't actually deal with the real problem. There is also the situation where a doctor assumes that their patient must be very sexually active when in fact they are not. This can cause a lot embarrassment for the patient and can easily damage the relationship between them. It can make some women far too embarrassed to seek further treatment at a later date.

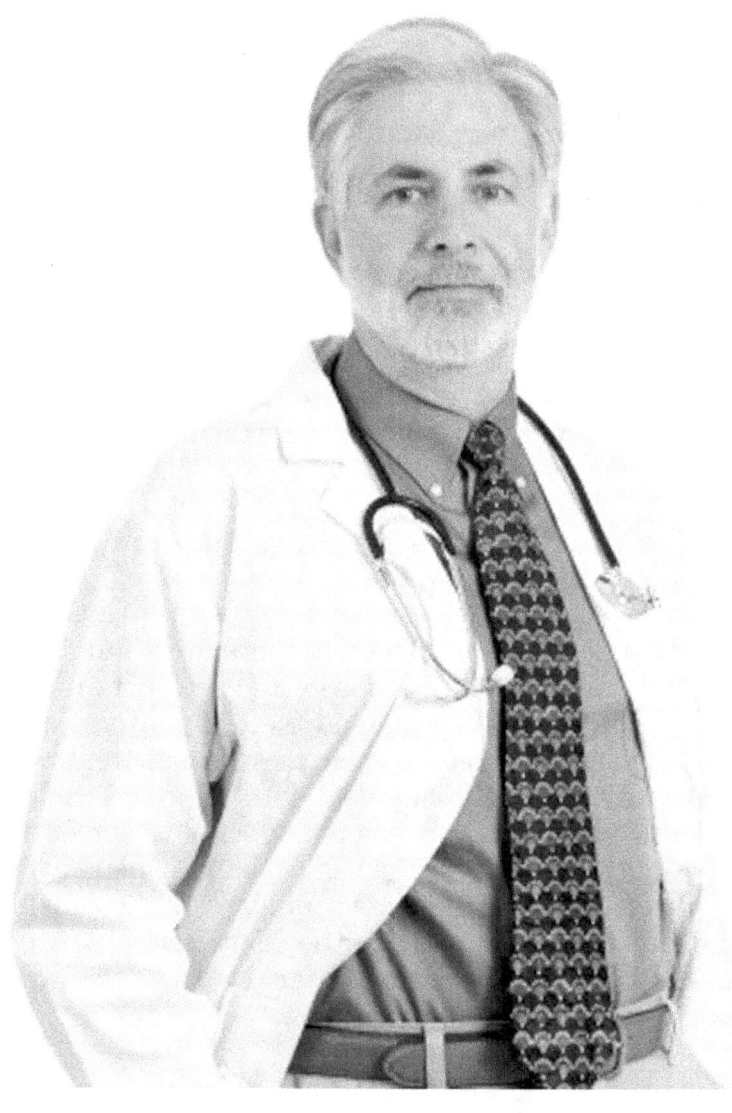

Male doctors can be the least sensitive about the problems caused by bacterial vaginosis. They either don't see this as an important condition or think that the women have to make the choices about lifestyle changes in order to deal with the infection.

Another problem is that doctors can have particular medicines that they prescribe for all vaginal infections. These antibiotics may be great for most uses, but they can often be excessive for treating bacterial vaginosis. If the drug choices doctors make are not well targeted to the condition they can overload the system and cause a lot of damage to the good bacteria that are important for the balance in the vaginal environment.

Like it or not doctors are influenced by the pharmaceutical companies that supply the drugs that they use. As a result they often push the use of such things as antibiotics in order to sell more products. This in turn can alter the way that doctors view the treatment of certain conditions such as bacterial vaginosis. It is easy to see that bacterial vaginosis can be a profit winner for them due to the chronic nature of the condition and the need for repeated and varied antibiotic treatments for individual women. This may mean that patients have to get their doctor round to the idea of alternative treatments as part of the mix in controlling their bacterial vaginosis.

Conditions That Make Bacterial Vaginosis Worse

Some existing conditions that women have can end up making bacterial vaginosis worse. In these circumstances it can be harder to manage and harder to cure.

Chronic yeast infection

Yeast infections set up the ideal conditions for the development of bacterial vaginosis in the way that it changes the balance of good and bad bacteria in the vagina. Even treating yeast infections is a problem as the drugs used will also wipe out bacterial growths whether they are the bad ones or the good ones. This in itself can cause problems as we saw earlier with antibiotic treatments.

Low estrogen hormone levels

When the estrogen hormone levels are lower than normal, the lining of the vagina becomes thinner and as a result it is more liable to infection.

High estrogen hormone levels

The main reasons for estrogen levels being higher than normal is due to taking contraceptive pills. Pregnancy is another reason for higher levels. Higher estrogen levels go hand in hand with a larger risk of bacterial infection. In the case of pregnancy treatments have to be sensitive to the health of the developing baby.

Allergies

All allergies can be a problem because they affect the way that the immune system reacts to conditions within the body. However, women who have allergies to certain antibiotic treatments can have their options for dealing with bacterial vaginosis severely limited. The stronger antibiotics needed for advanced treatment of bacterial vaginosis may not be tolerated by a woman with allergies to antibiotics and as a result they are left with only alternative therapies to choose from

Autoimmune disease

Autoimmune type conditions can reduce the body's ability to deal with infections. This can give rise to bacterial vaginosis infections going unchecked and resulting in chronic infections that are very difficult to deal with. Autoimmune diseases include HIV and Lupus.

Bacterial Vaginosis and Menstruation

Changes during menstruation can lead to an episode of bacterial vaginosis. Hormonal changes in particular have been identified with the start of bacterial vaginosis. During scientific research studying vaginal smears it has been found that the bad bacteria begin to grow during the follicular stage of the menstrual cycle. This is during the first 17 days of the cycle when estrogen levels are high.

When blood is released during menstruation this can also be a time for an increase in bacterial vaginosis. It is thought that this is due to the fact that blood has a pH of around 7.4 and this means that blood present in the vagina will increase the overall pH which is more favorable to the growth of bacterial vaginosis bacteria.

When the menstrual cycle stops during pregnancy it has been found that bacterial vaginosis will simply disappear in fifty percent of women. This is probably due to the fact that levels of the hormone progesterone start to rise at this time.

You should note any changes in your period as this can be an indication that a bacterial vaginosis infection is involved. Here are some of the changes that could be associated with bacterial vaginosis:

Having heavier periods
Longer periods which last up to 7 days
Blood clots or lumps of blood that are very noticeable
Thicker menstrual blood
More mucus in the blood
Later starting periods
Earlier starting periods
Missing periods

Bacterial vaginosis can lead to more serious conditions and as a result if you notice any of the above changes to your period after an episode of bacterial vaginosis you should get it checked out just in case. Excessive blood clots could be a sign of polyp formation in the uterus which could cause problems during pregnancy including miscarriages. If in doubt always seek further medical advice.

Bacterial Vaginosis in Pregnancy

Even a pregnant woman can get bacterial vaginosis, which becomes a risk for the unborn child as well as the mother if left untreated. According to the Centers for Disease Control, Bacterial Vaginosis is found in over one million pregnant women, more than Herpes, Chlamydia or other sexually transmitted diseases.

Bacterial vaginosis during pregnancy is not unusual. The American Pregnancy Association reports that 10% to 30% of women have bacterial vaginosis during the course of their pregnancies. That shatters the myth that bacterial vaginosis cannot be contracted during pregnancy.

Unless a woman reports bacterial vaginosis type symptoms, many doctors do not screen for this infection. Women need to be pro-active for their health and that of their unborn child by insisting that the doctor conducts bacterial vaginosis screening as a precaution.

Bacteria have a nasty habit of spreading so when a pregnant woman has bacterial vaginosis, the bacteria can move into the womb or fallopian tubes. At that point, the bacteria become an infection known as pelvic inflammatory disease (PID). Left untreated, PID is a leading cause of infertility as well as ectopic pregnancy.

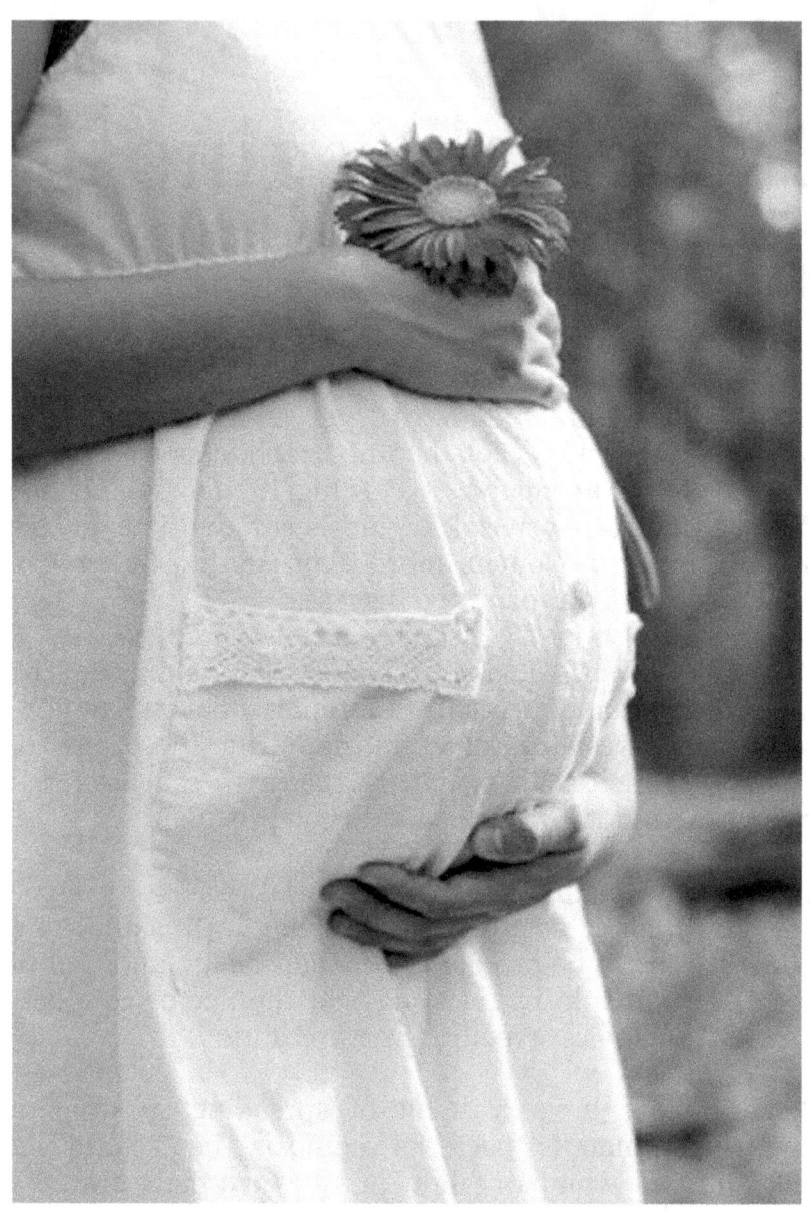

Another risk factor for pregnant women who have bacterial vaginosis is premature delivery or a baby with low birth weight. The Centers for Disease Control (CDC) recommend that any woman with a history of low birth weight babies or premature delivery needs to be tested for bacterial vaginosis early in their next pregnancy.

There are antibiotic treatments that can be taken by many pregnant women without harm to the baby. The choice of antibiotics needs to be left to the Obstetrician who knows the woman's overall health and determine potential risks to the unborn baby.

Bacterial Vaginosis and Infertility

Women who want to get pregnant but are not conceiving begin to search aggressively for the problem. If all the basic equipment for conception and carrying a baby are intact, then the fertility specialist begins to look for other conditions that can be treated.

Pelvic Inflammatory Disease (PID) is a condition that is on the rise among women of childbearing age. PID can so drastically damage the fallopian tubes and uterus that pregnancy is impossible or if pregnancy occurs, the danger for ectopic pregnancy is extreme. When the egg gets trapped in a fallopian tube that is damaged or twisted from infection, the pregnancy will not develop. If left undetected, the tube will eventually burst from the pressure of the growing egg.

There is usually no warning that what is assumed to be a normal pregnancy is actually an ectopic pregnancy. So when the tube ruptures immediate medical care is necessary. This type of miscarriage can also be life threatening to the mother.

What many women don't know is that Bacterial Vaginosis is an infection, which left untreated, can lead to the development of Pelvic Inflammatory Disease. This is a serious medical problem. The irritating bacterial vaginosis symptoms that seem to interfere with an active social life in younger ages may be the death knell to the dream of having a healthy baby a few years later if PID causes permanent damage to the reproductive system.

This dangerous connection with PID is another reason that bacterial vaginosis cannot be ignored or taken lightly. Once PID sets in, a woman is not just at risk of infertility but also for other serious medical consequences.

Bacterial Vaginosis and Sex

Some women believe that sexual intercourse with their partner can start off a bout of bacterial vaginosis. It has even been suggested that the sperm form some men can act as a contributory factor. The one sure thing is that sexual intercourse can cause the infection to get worse. As a result women may abstain from sex during the time that they have the infection. The main thing is to get to know your own body and how it reacts to bacterial vaginosis during times of sexual intercourse.

Because bacterial vaginosis creeps up before the serious symptoms signal the presence of the infection, women are often involved in an active sex life as bacterial vaginosis is developing. For some women, it's a comment from a partner about the fishy odor or the sticky discharge that alerts them to the problem if no other symptoms are felt.

When bacterial vaginosis mixes with semen, it produces the kind of horrible smell produced from a chemical reaction that cleared the chemistry lab in high school. This situation can be embarrassing and lead to a shy goodbye.

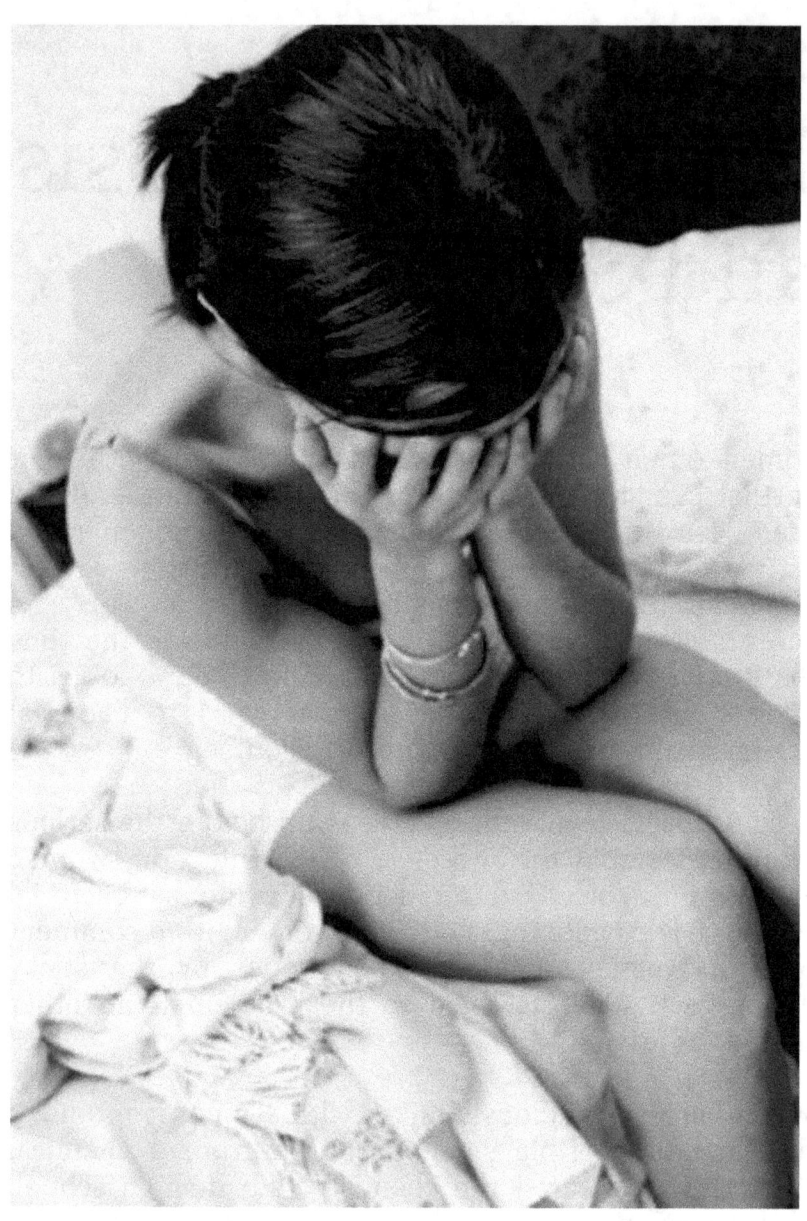

Who can feel sexy and alluring knowing that once the clothes come off, the partner may be turned off by the foul smelling vaginal discharge? Just the fear of being rejected because of bacterial vaginosis is enough to test a relationship.

Explaining the bacterial vaginosis condition is taking the honest approach, which may or may not be well received. Some women are concerned that to even admitting to a vaginal infection will cause the partner to think that it's really something worse such as HIV and shun them.

Another real turn-off is when a woman makes repeated trips to the bathroom in an effort to wash away the discharge or add perfumed lotions to counteract the bacterial vaginosis   smell that distracts from the moment. The worst idea is to use scented vaginal lubricants as a way to mask the foul odor from the bacterial vaginosis. It's like attempting to camouflage the smell of burned food with a floral spray. The mixture is totally disgusting and even worse than the initial bad smell.

As an infection, bacterial vaginosis   causes the vagina to be tender, stretched and uncomfortable with vaginal intercourse. Faking an orgasm is one thing, but faking enjoyment when the entire vaginal area is as irritated as a third degree sunburn isn't happening. Talk about ruining the romantic scene, the symptoms of bacterial vaginosis can certainly do that.

Bacterial Vaginosis in Men

It has always been thought that men are not associated with bacterial vaginitis and as a result it isn't anything that they should be concerned with. However, there seem to be a number of women who disagree and strongly believe that their partner is re-infecting them in some way. The importance of this is that women have to ask themselves whether their partner should be treated for the infection as well

In considering this situation it is important to understand that the male reproductive system is fundamentally different to the female one. As a result the conditions do not exist within it to encourage the vigorous growth of the organisms associated with bacterial vaginosis, as seen in women. As a result the bacteria cannot grow. However, despite this men may carry other types of bacteria which can be passed onto the woman during sexual intercourse.

Although there is no medical proof it is possible that men may have traces of the BV bacteria in their urethra tube and as a result reinfection could be caused in this way. Men show no symptoms of bacterial vaginosis although the bacteria may be present within the reproductive system. For this reason some doctors are sympathetic to women who keep getting re-infected and may suggest treating the male partner as well even if this is to eliminate them from being the cause of the reinfections.

Even if you believe that men are not responsible for reinfections you have to consider the fact that sperm from men does appear to make existing infections worse. The reaction between the semen and the infection within the woman often causes the release of a strong smell. This in itself may lead women to think that the man is re-infecting them even though it may just be identifying an existing low level infection within the woman.

The possibility of treating both partners for bacterial vaginosis is something that needs to be discussed between sexually active partners and their individual doctors. This could in itself be a tricky conversation.

Bacterial Vaginosis and Surgery

During any kind of surgery there is always the risk of infection. This means that any surgery in the area of the vagina could set up the conditions for developing bacterial vaginosis later on. In addition, if a woman already has a mild case of bacterial vaginosis then, the surgery can then exacerbate the problem.

Bacterial vaginosis testing should be requested during pregnancy if there is the slightest chance of a Caesarean section having to take place. Expectant mothers have to think about this early on because emergency Caesarean sections tend to come around really quickly towards the end of pregnancy.

Abortion is another area where bacterial vaginosis could cause problems. It has been shown that it can become a risk in post abortion recovery. Any operation that involves the female reproductive organs poses a risk and this includes such things as hysterectomy. In all of these cases it is important that a test for bacterial vaginosis is done.

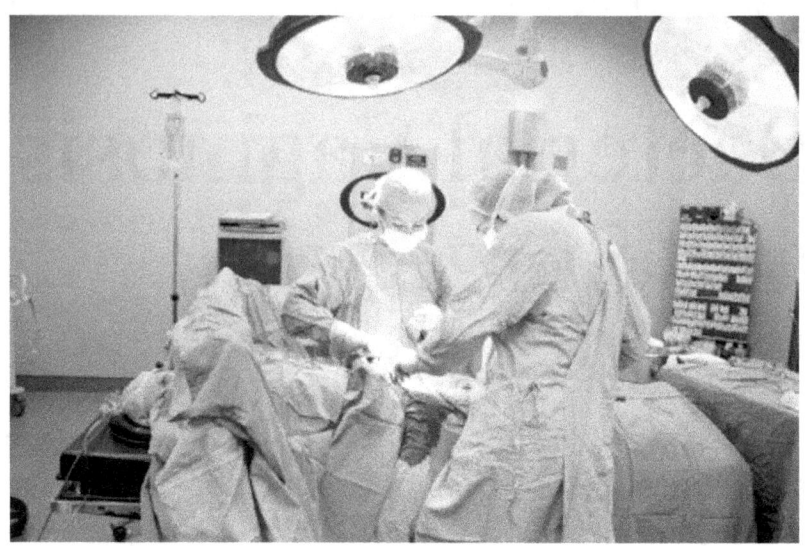

If you are going in for surgery you should never ignore the symptoms of bacterial vaginosis. Don't think that it will be something that will just go away on its own. The infection can easily become worse and this can delay your recovery from any surgery that you have undertaken. Ultimately, the infection could make any post-operative problems worse and it could actually become life threatening in extreme cases.

Bacterial Vaginosis Freedom

Preventing Bacterial Vaginosis

It stands to reason that the best way to deal with bacterial vaginosis is not to get it in the first place. If you've had bacterial vaginosis before, you certainly won't want to get it again. In order to prevent infection and reinfection you really have to look at your life style and make changes that will reduce the chances of it all happening again.

None of the following suggestions are difficult or even expensive. Mainly it is simply a case of becoming aware of conditions in which bacterial vaginosis thrives and then deciding on and making other choices.

When women become proactive about their health, they are in control of their bodies and not dependent on drugs or doctors to solve the problem. It is therefore better to avoid infection than deal with curing it. This isn't to imply that infection prevention is easy. However, a few basic precautions go a long way to protecting a woman from bacterial vaginosis or from a reoccurrence of the condition. Here are some suggestions for actions that you can take:

Reduce or stop douching. Even liquids made for douche are strong enough to upset the balance of good bacteria to bad bacteria. Douching can actually make bacterial vaginosis worse. A strong douche can cause newly forming bacterial vaginosis to spread further up the reproductive tract than it otherwise would.

Reduce the potential for E.coli bacteria from the rectum to enter the vagina by wiping from front to back after bowel movements.

Scented toilet paper may leave a nice smell in the bathroom, but the chemicals in the scent can irritate the vaginal area. It is therefore best to use unscented toilet paper.

Personal hygiene products with scents of fruits or flowers are advertised as sexy but the perfume within the product can be too harsh for the vaginal area. Once again these are best avoided.

Clean up after sex. Forget the lingering moment and think about how the moisture and semen are a breeding ground for bacteria. Wash gently with an antibacterial cleanser, which is made for use in the vaginal area Do not just whatever soap is handy at the time.

Classic white cotton panties may not be a fashionable as a lace thong but they are less likely to allow the growth of bacteria. Cotton is a natural fiber that absorbs moisture and allows for air circulation. You should keep several pairs available for normal wear.

Women who use diaphragms or cervical caps must wash these carefully, rinse and dry before using them again. These devices not only prevent pregnancy but the tight fit creates an ideal place for bacterial growth if they are not properly cleaned before use.

Always practice safe sex. The use of condoms is important to reduce the spread of STD's or other infections between partners.

Keeping Dry

Wearing wet clothes can contribute to the development of Bacterial Vaginosis. Think about how many times you come out of the pool and laze on the patio sunbathing in a wet swimsuit. The tendency is to remain in your swimsuit because it is convenient. After all, why dry off and get dressed when you might want to get back into the water? It is better to change into clean dry clothes, rinse out the swim suit and let it dry before putting it on again. Even the best cleaned pool is still a place that bacteria can grow.

In a lake, it is even worse for bacterial vaginosis infection and many other infections. Swimming in a lake or stream may seem like harmless fun, but a few days later when the bacterial vaginosis symptoms start you will realize that the fun is definitely over.

If you regularly go swimming, water skiing, diving or snorkeling you should bring two or three swimsuits and extra dry towels to change rather than let your wet swimsuit become a breeding ground for bacteria. You should remember that a little extra laundry is much easier to manage than bacterial vaginosis.

Towels are another problem that is often overlooked. This is can be challenging because even hotels put out signs asking that guests reuse towels to save water. Being environmentally friendly is all very well but you also have to manage your vaginal environment, which does not need repeated infection. Using a towel again that has already been damp is another error that women can make. Take a beach towel to sit on but use a fresh, clean towel to dry your body.

Women who have had repeated episodes of bacterial vaginosis know the importance of drying the vaginal area before getting dressed. Some women find that using the hair dryer on a low setting is better for drying the vulva area than causing new irritations to the delicate tissue by rubbing with a towel.

Underwear

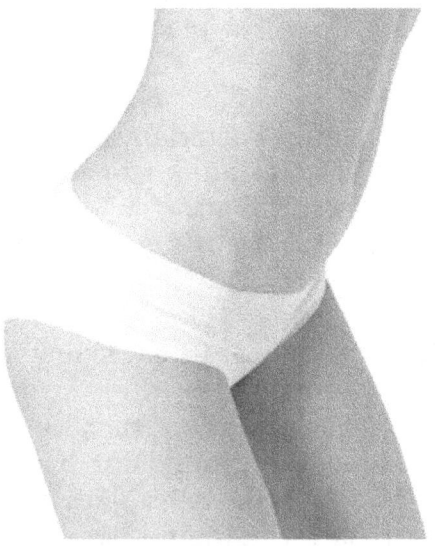

Wearing clean underwear every day is vital to your vaginal health. Try not to become lazy by getting out of bed at the last possible minute and then throwing on your clothes in order to rush off to work

Even if you are a last minute dresser or if you want to wait until after work to take a long soak in the bath, you still need to change underwear. Make sure you put on clean panties either before going to bed at night or when getting dressed in the morning.

Anytime you wear pantyhose or tights, make certain to wash these after every use. It is also better to avoid wearing these during an outbreak of bacterial vaginosis. Pantyhose and tights literally encase you from legs to waist. Even in colder weather, your body temperature warms when you are inside a building. This is when this warm, secluded area becomes ideal for bacterial infection growth. It is fine to wear pantyhose or tights without panties but you should treat them the same as you do panties and wash them after every wear.

Sexy underwear tends to be alluring but not the best choice for keeping infection at a distance. Save the sexy underwear for the right place and time and wear the cotton panties at other times, especially if you have an outbreak of bacterial vaginosis or have just finished one. Cotton panties may not be sexy to your partner, but neither is the fishy odor of bacterial vaginosis.

Washing Clothes

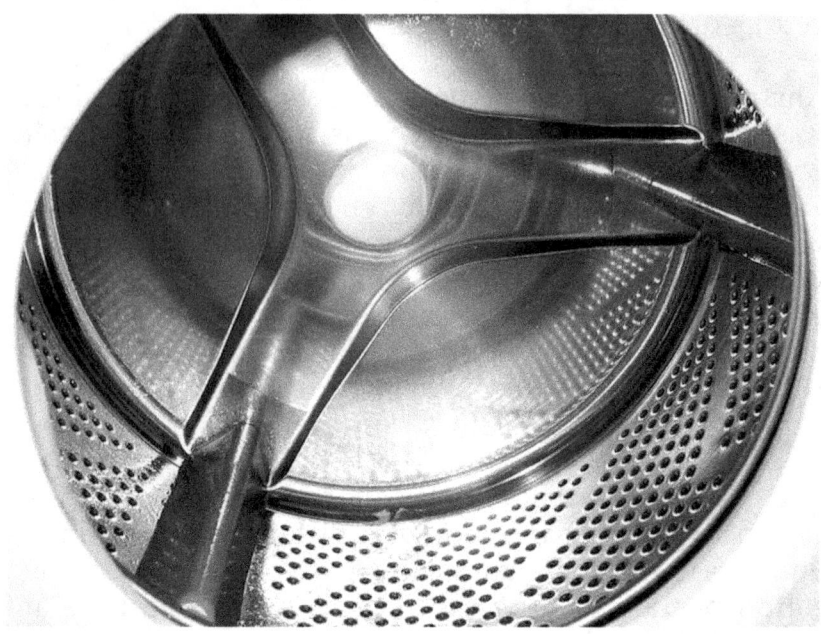

A lot of people just throw all of their washing into the machine without sorting it. This is a bad idea. Separating your clothes for different wash cycles, detergents and temperatures not only increases the useful life of clothing, but also allows you to regulate the use of chemicals that could affect your body.

Hypoallergenic laundry detergent is essential for women who are susceptible to bacterial infections. You should choose one that is fragrance free. As nice as the spring breeze smell might be, a better way to get that fresh smell is by hanging your sheets and towels on the line to dry than by adding a version of chemical sunshine.

There is no need to go over the top with bleach in the wash. Wash bath towels, swim towel and wash cloths in fragrance free, hypoallergenic detergent at a hot water setting and then place them in the dryer straight away. Leaving wet towels to linger in the washing machine before drying is one more breeding opportunity for bacteria.

A lot of modern washing machines have a drum made of plastic rather than the stainless steel that was used in the past. This is specially so for cheaper machines. Even if the drum is made from stainless steel the casing will be plastic. This type of drum has lots of nooks and crannies where bacteria can grow. You may have noticed that the machine will start to smell when it is left idle, especially if the door has been left closed. The smell is caused by the growth of bacteria and fungi in the machine. Unless you deal with this situation the bacteria and fungi will be transferred to your clothes during the time that your clothes are being washed. This is bad news if you are expecting to put clean clothes on because they will be covered with these bacteria that are only going to make the problems of bacterial vaginosis worse. To deal with this problem, make sure that you do a maintenance wash every month using no clothes and a detergent containing bleach at the highest temperature that your machine will allow. You can also add a couple of spoons of sodium bicarbonate to each wash in order to keep the levels of bacteria in your machine as low as possible.

Bubble Bath

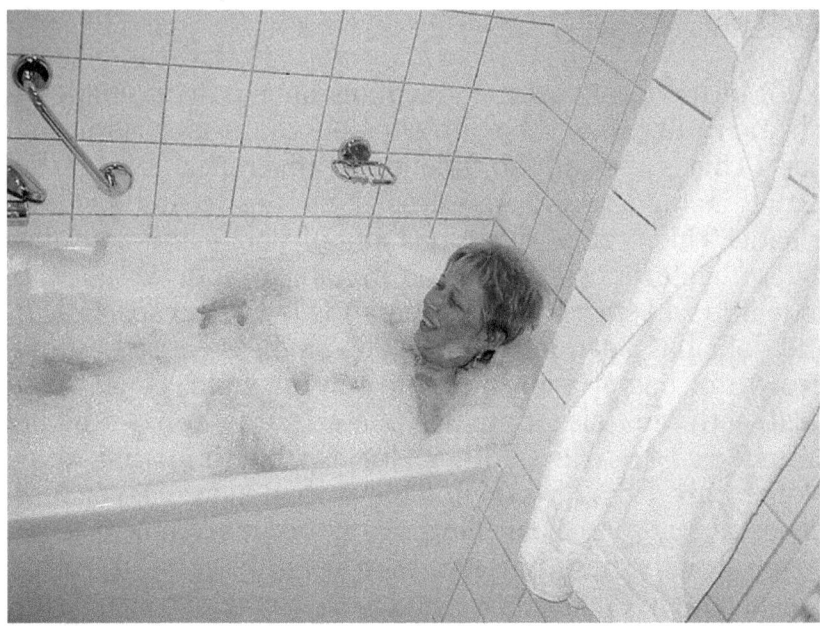

No matter how much you want a long soak in a hot bubble bath after a hard day at work, this is not the best thing to do during or straight after an episode of bacterial vaginosis. The chemicals in bubble bath can be too strong for an already aggravated vaginal area. When a bacterial vaginosis episode is at its peak, you will feel a harsh stinging sensation and this will make you get out of the bath very quickly indeed. However, if the bacterial vaginosis infection is just beginning and has yet to produce major symptoms then, although, you will feel no stinging the long soak will just encourage the infection.

Use a natural soap without added fragrances for washing your skin. One that is recommended for the delicate skin of babies is a good choice. Other soaps include the basic soaps like 'Ivory soap' from the supermarket or organic soaps from the health food shop.

Sharing Things

Although sharing is something to be encouraged, when it comes to bacterial vaginosis it is definitely a bad idea.

Partners should not share bath towels. If you had an athlete's foot infection then you would definitely not share towels and the problem of bacterial vaginosis is no different to this. The idea here is to stop infections being passed around within the family. What you spread will come round again and get you back.

A good idea is to get his and her towels. These could simply be different colors. In this way you will definitely know which one is yours. An alternative is to keep the two sets of towels in different palaces. You have to be consistent with this and make sure that your partner doesn't simply use yours because they are closer to hand.

When women are experiencing a bacterial vaginosis episode, it is best not to wipe the vulva with a bath towel as the typical washing machine is not a sterile machine. Another option is to use disposable soft cloths or buy a set of cheap small washcloths that are only used for this purpose.

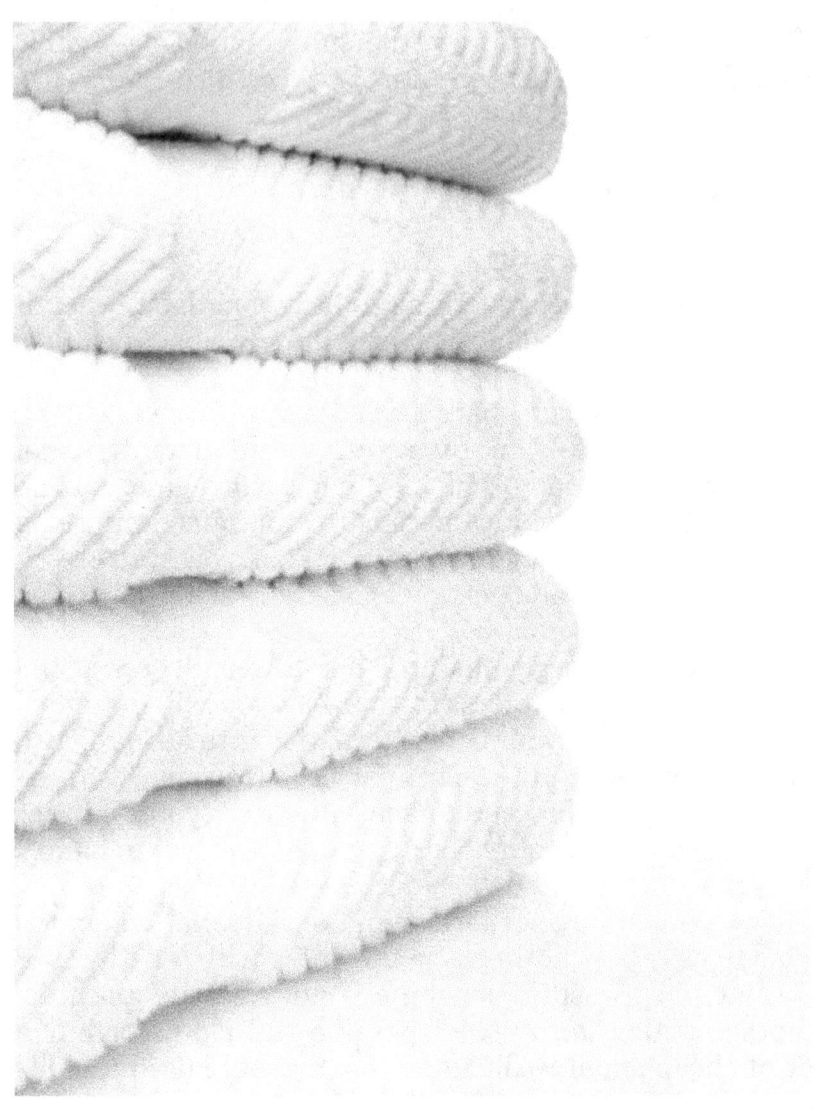

Stop it Coming Back Again

The immune system is designed to protect you from infections and when it is working correctly it can deal with the odd flare up associated with bacterial vaginosis. One problem is that if the immune system is busy fighting lots of other things it may become so stressed and stretched that it can't cope in the fight against the latest assault from the bacteria vaginosis infection. As a result, it makes sense to not only keep your immune system in tip top condition but also to try and reduce the amount of stress that it is under.

Typically the immune system has to deal with the infective organisms and the toxins that they produce. It also has to deal with any other toxins that get into the body. Toxins can come from inside the body as waste products and from outside as external factors such as pollution. It stands to reason that all of these toxins put a strain on the immune system. The best thing would be to avoid them, and therefore knowing where they come from is a good start in trying to protect your immune system.

Here are some lists of common toxins that your body may encounter. You can use the lists to decide which ones that you are exposed to on a regular basis

Typical toxins in the environment

Air pollution
Auto exhaust fumes
Pesticides
Fertilizers
Ozone
Pollen

Perfumes
Cleaning liquids
Chlorine for pool cleaning
Dust Mite waste
Cigarette and cigar smoke
Smoke from outdoor leaf burning or forest fires
Construction or demolition sites

Typical toxins inside the body

Alcohol
Illegal drug use
Prescription drug abuse
Food coloring
Food stabilizers
Food emulsifiers
Food additives and preservative
Cigarette and cigar smoking
Mold
Parasites
Metal in the body (screws, plates, dental work)
Tampons
Hair dye
Cosmetics
Hormone imbalance
Free radicals

You should produce a plan to reduce your exposure to these types of toxins. This could include:

Removing the toxins from your home and work place

Reduce your exposure to the toxins that you can't eliminate

Substitute safer alternatives where elimination causes problems

Each toxin that you manage to remove or avoid gives your immune system a better chance when it comes to fighting bacterial vaginosis. This should make it less likely that you will suffer from recurring infections.

One way of dealing with toxins that are already in the body is to use a suitable detoxification method:

Using a Detox Patch

A detox patch is usually put on the bottom of the feet just before you go to bed and left to do its magic overnight. The active ingredients of a detox patch are designed to deal with various toxins and are produced by alternative medicine practitioners. The way that the patch works is that it draws out toxins from the body and then they are taken up by the patch which is later discarded. As the detox process takes place while you are sleeping, this is an easy to use method of detoxification.

Detox Recipes

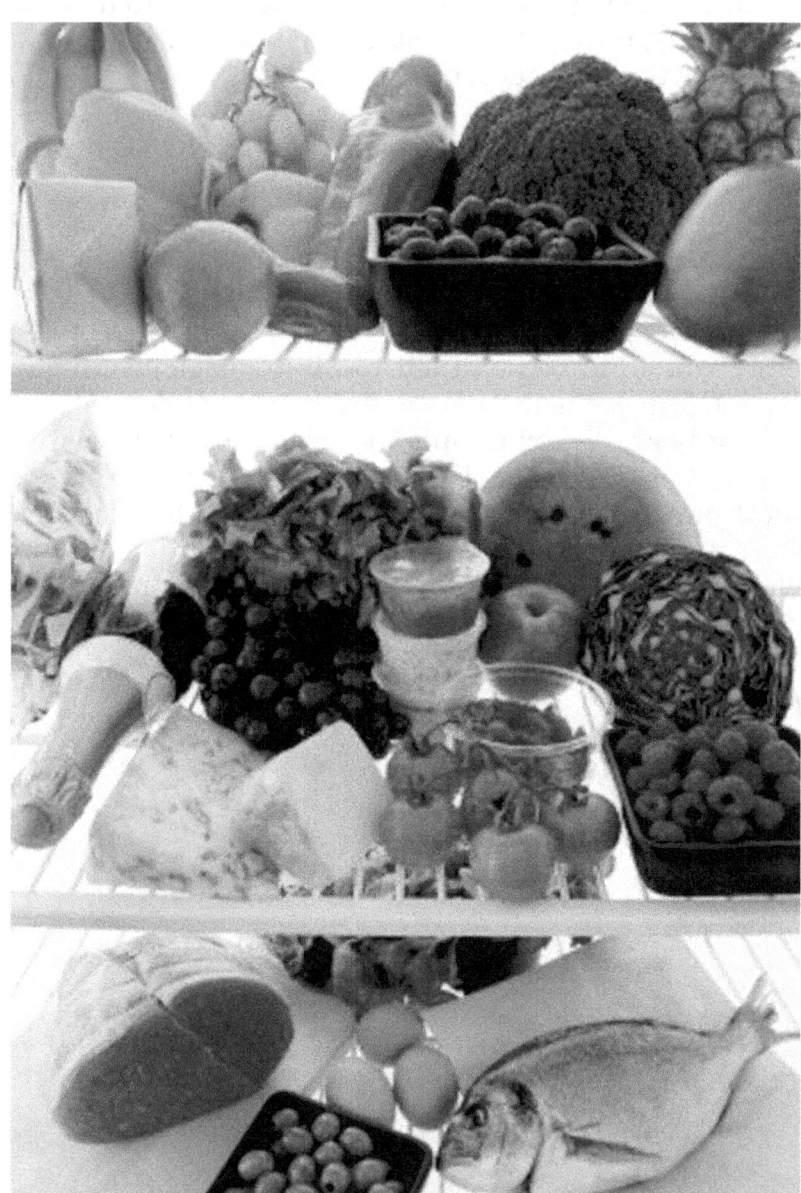

These are particular foods that build up the body's immune system using fresh ingredients and high quality proteins. You can get a cookbook that explains how to buy and put together detox menus. It will also tell you how to stock your refrigerator with healthy foods that build up your body and help it fight the organisms that cause bacterial vaginosis. Even if you are busy working and commuting you should be able to produce at least one meal using detox recipes. On the weekends when you have more time you can make sure that you increase your intake of detox foods. One easy way to produce detox foods is in the form of a green smoothie.

Green Smoothie Detox

Green smoothies could be part of a detox program, if that is what you want, but it is better to change over to a more natural green smoothie diet all of the time. If you are already taking green smoothies on a regular basis they will be doing their job all of the time and removing any toxins.

Toxins or poisonous substances are usually introduced by bad habits such as poor diets or smoking cigarettes. These toxins are usually in the form of chemicals which end up producing free radicals which can damage cells. The magic ingredients for dealing with these free radicals and chemicals are antioxidants. Fruits and vegetables are full of these health giving antioxidants so green smoothies are a great choice if detoxing is what you want to do. You should remember that any detoxing that you do will not be helped if you are still on a poor diet.

When you make your detox smoothies try to select fruits and vegetables with high levels of antioxidants and vitamins. Vitamin C is a good choice and fruits are a natural choice. Use spring water, if you can, as it won't contain chemicals like chlorine. You could even use Rooibos or green tea instead as these both contain lots of antioxidants. Rooibos is probably the better choice because it has the advantage of having no tannins or caffeine in it. It is better to drink Rooibos tea throughout the day and avoid such things as sport drinks, alcohol and sodas. Drinking a lot of this tea or pure water will help to purge your body of toxins as they will be excreted via the kidneys together with the water. The extra water will make you go more often. You should also make sure that you get enough sleep during your detox regime as well. Sleep gives the body a chance to recover and repair itself.

Detoxing using green smoothies will soon have you feeling better as the toxins are removed from your body. As well as this you will feel like you have extra energy and your thinking will become easier and your mind more relaxed.

All green smoothies are good for detox but you can boost their effect by choosing fruits and vegetables that have a particular profile. Adding more fruits will increase the amount of vitamin C which is essential for a good detox. Potassium can be increased by adding more banana, and blueberries are very good as a source of antioxidants. Beta carotene is found in carrots and this is also good to have in a detox smoothie. All you need to do is decide which part of your detox that you are aiming at and increase the amount of a fruit or vegetable that supply the right active ingredient.

The recipe below is a popular one that is often used in detox regimes:

1 ½ cups of cold Rooibos or green tea
1 romaine lettuce
3 celery stalks
2 apples
1 banana
1/3 bunch of coriander
1/3 bunch of parsley

Juice of 1/2 a fresh lemon

This particular green smoothie works well at detoxing the liver. This is important because many important metabolic reactions occur in the liver including those used to detoxify poisons. A well-functioning liver is reflected in the general health of the body. Coriander helps to deal with heavy metals, if they are in the body. Heavy metals can disrupt important metabolic reactions. The fresh fruit contains many vitamins which often get depleted when the body is run down and having to deal with toxic substances. As well as this it is loaded with antioxidants to deal with free radicals which cause cells to prematurely age. The best way to take your smoothie is as a large glass every morning as part of a general cleansing of the body.

Besides having your usual green smoothies each day you can also go for a detox smoothie at the start of each week. This sets you up ready for the week to come. This could be better for you than just having detox purges. Here is a recipe for one such weekly detox smoothie:

Flesh of 1 lemon
2 pears
2 apples
3 tbsp flax oil
½ tsp of turmeric
¼ tsp of course sea salt
Pinch of cayenne pepper
4 cups cold fresh water

This is a truly remarkable detox recipe which is ideal to have as breakfast on a Monday morning. The lemon and flax oil are really good at detoxifying the liver and at the same time they will help your immune system to work correctly. This is due to the extra Vitamin C and omega 3 fatty acids that they provide. The added turmeric is good for the blood and skin. This smoothie will boost your energy levels, which is just the thing most people need on a Monday morning before they have to trudge off to work. If you like the effects of this smoothie then you could have it more than once a week so that all of your important organ systems are kicked into top gear.

Here are some more detoxifying green smoothies that you can try and integrate into your weekly regime:

Down under detox

2 cups green grapes
3 kiwi fruits
1 medium orange
2 tbsp of Aloe Vera juice
6 leaves romaine lettuce
2 cups cold fresh water

Tropical delight

1 romaine lettuce
1 handful of parsley
½ avocado
Juice of 1 lime
2 cups of coconut water
2 tsp of honey

Caribbean garden detox

½ bunch dandelion greens
½ inch fresh ginger root
2 ripe peaches
½ ripe pineapple
Fresh cold water

Detox Bath

Once you have your bacterial vaginosis infection under control getting into a detox bath can be a rather pleasant preventative. You can treat yourself to a detox bath at a luxurious day spa to start off with. During this time you can learn how to create a detox bath for yourself.

Detox baths can be replicated at home and you can use your own cozy bathrobe and candles to really set the scene. You can use some simple kinds of ingredients that can be bought at the local supermarket health food shop. Here are the things you need:

1 cup sea salt
1 cup Epsom salt
2 cups baking soda

Simply mix up the dry ingredients in a bowl and then slowly add these to the water as the bath is fills up. This is the best way to mix the salt mixture with the water. You can make multiple amounts of the dry mixture and keep it in a tightly closed glass jars ready for the next time.

Make sure that the water temperature is kept warm not hot. Epsom salt will encourage sweating which helps the body's natural ways of removing toxins. You should note that when taken together a hot bath and Epsom salt can be dangerous for a people who have high blood pressure, diabetes or heart disease. You should seek medical advice if you are unsure about this.

Colon Detox

In addition to body detoxification you can also try a colon is detoxification. The easiest way to do this is with a 7 or 10 day colon cleansing kit which you can obtain from a health food store or alternative medicine shop. Make sure that you follow the directions that come with the kit.

While the colon cleansing is taking place follow the recommended food and drink intake precisely. After cleansing you should replenish the good bacteria with probiotic yogurt and acidophilus dairy products or supplements.

While you may feel tired as colon cleansing takes place, you will later experience a big energy surge when the body has got rid of the excess waste and toxins.

When the colon is working at its best, the body eliminates waste daily so that bacteria loses another important breeding area. Adding more fiber to your food choices is the way to improve colon action. Fiber is also more filling than other food so you need less to feel full.

Another way to get good colon health is simply to drink more water. The 8 glasses of water recommended for good general health are also important to wash out the colon and provide smooth movement for food through the intestines. Nutrients are then absorbed more easily and waste products discarded more efficiently. A lot of women who have recurrent bacterial vaginosis have been found to also have chronic constipation and this is a symptom of poor colon health.

Liver Detox

The liver is the central hard working organ of your body that gets to deal daily with pollutants, medications, caffeine, smoke and other internal toxins. It chemically removes these toxins from your body as well as regulating the energy levels of your body. If you add to this the poor quality of the typical Western diet and the workload of the liver is great

Select a liver detox kit from the health shop or alternative medicine center. The method is like that used for the colon cleanse. The only caution is that you cannot do these simultaneously. You need to complete the colon cleanse and wait the amount of time recommended on the product before starting the liver cleanse.

Detoxification of the body is not a one-time event that lasts forever. This is because toxins continually attack the body and as a result you need to make detoxification procedures an ongoing part of your approach to healthy living.

Producing a Plan

When you are suffering with Bacterial Vaginosis symptoms all you can think of is how you would do almost anything to get some relief from it. You will find that you will try to get information and actions to take from almost anywhere and then there are all of the Doctor's appointments as well.

With a lot less effort, you can start to plan a bacterial vaginosis free lifestyle. This means that instead of frantically trying to find a cure, you will be setting up the conditions that eliminate the recurrence of bacterial vaginosis.

To get good results you need to plan and monitor what you are doing. Take another look at the list of internal and external toxins given above. Make two copies of this page to use in your evaluation.

Choose the main five internal toxins to which you are regularly exposed and list each in a table with the headings given below. Rate your progress in dealing with these internal toxins as 'Improved' or 'Needs Improvement'.

Internal Toxin

Improved

Needs Improvement

Action Plan

For each item that you rated as 'needs improvement' list a few ideas in the Action Plan section for how your will deal with this toxin. The action plan might include:

Obtaining more information or research
Consulting with an alternative medicine practitioner or nutritionist
Eliminating unhealthy habits with a stop smoking program or weight loss plan

The action plan must only ideas that you produce and that you are willing to actually do something about. This is not a wish list or a goals list. This is an Action Plan, which means you have to put some action to the words otherwise nothing will change.

Next you should repeat the process by selecting the top five external toxins to which you are regularly exposed and list each in a table using the headings given below. Rate your progress in dealing with these internal toxins as 'Improved' or 'Needs Improvement'.

External Toxins

Improved

Needs Improvement

Action Plan

For each item that you rated as "needs improvement," list a few ideas in the Action Plan for how your will deal with this toxin.

The action plan might include such things as:

Changing your transportation method
More frequent change of air system filters in your home,
Avoiding restaurants and public places where there is exposure to second hand smoke
Changing from pesticides to natural methods for outdoor and indoor plants

Sleep and Stress

Women who have bacterial vaginosis tend to be very busy people. These are typically productive workers, professionals, mothers and students who are always multi-tasking and working to their limit. When being too busy becomes normality the extra pressure puts a strain on their physical and emotional health. Both of these can harm the immune system's ability to fight infection.

The important things that need balancing out are stress and sleep. To live a bacterial vaginosis free life, women have to pay a lot of attention to these important issues. Stress has been well researched and has been identified as a pre-condition for bacterial vaginosis. A body that is under constant stress abuses the hormonal system with repeated pressure to go beyond reasonable limits. Women can seem to be living on adrenaline. This results in stress that is very is negative. This type of stress can lead to headaches, irritability, high blood pressure, strokes, car and industrial accidents. There is simply nothing good or useful about this sort of stress. Positive stress is the kind that is more like anticipation or excitement such as the way you feel getting married, starting college, becoming a new mother, starting the first day of a new job or signing the deeds for your first home. This kind of stress is only short lived and is very manageable.

There is of course negative stress that happens as part of a normal life style. This is often when it is least expected. It comes on quickly, is dealt with and then goes away. Here you don't get the chance to fret over everything. Learning to manage stress is very important when it comes to living a bacterial vaginosis free life.

Sleep deprivation is a serious problem for a lot of women. Many women are stressed with so much to do that they often stay up late and get up early. Four or five hours sleep a day and trying to make up for it at weekends just doesn't work. Sleep deprivation builds up over the days and nights and the damage to your body occurs a little more each day.

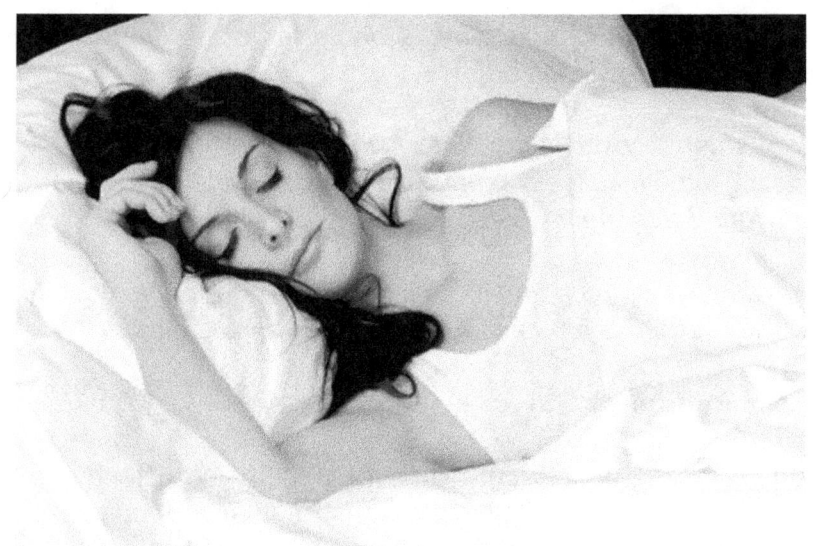

To keep healthy a woman needs 8-9 hours of sleep every night. This means that changes in lifestyle are needed:

Turn off the television, computer and cell phone at least half hour before bedtime.

Take a bath and relax before bedtime so your body can wind down from a busy day.

Don't go to sleep with the television or radio turned on.

If you want music, choose a CD with instrumental only, no vocals.

Establish a routine time for bed and time to get up in the morning.

Sleeping an extra hour on the weekend is fine just don't vary the times drastically. If you do, you make it harder to follow the sleep pattern when the workweek rolls around.

Avoid exercise, house cleaning, sports or other strenuous activities near bedtime.

Don't think that surfing the Internet is less strenuous. While you may be seated, your mind is running a marathon to keep up with all that input.

Shut down the laptop and make a rule not to work online while in bed. The bed is for sleeping and other intimate pursuits.

Become a Choosy Buyer

Bacterial Vaginosis symptoms can easily be affected by otherwise innocent appearing consumer products such as soaps and scents As a result you must become a choosy buyer by reading labels and ingredient lists so that you know what you are buying.

Make sure these chemicals aren't in your products:

Propylene glycol
Alcohol
Methyl benzethonium chloride
Artificial coloring
Sodium lauryl sulfate

Green products are also a good way to get more pure ingredients. Even so, you should still look at the labels just in case some of the ingredients might still be a problem.

Hypoallergenic and fragrance free products are designed to be kind to skin and these are just the sort of thing that you should be looking for. These products should be made from mainly natural ingredients and this is good for your body.

When it comes to sex using condoms is a good idea. It is best to buy the plain condoms that do not have a coating of spermicides, lubricants or fragrances. These substances could upset the balance of good bacteria to bad bacteria in the vagina. Natural lubricants should be used if there is a dryness during sex. These can be obtained from a health food store or alternative medicine center. Natural or organic products will provide the comfort you need without using chemicals you are trying to avoid.

Having a bacterial vaginosis free lifestyle is a woman's best defense against infections that could eventually result in serious problems such as Pelvic Inflammatory Disease. Women need to take control of their health decisions and avoid depending on prescription antibiotics. Antibiotics are not the answer to the problem whereas the prevention of bacterial vaginosis is the solution.

It is important to realize that by identifying and reducing or eliminating the internal and external toxins, taking good health precautions, using safe sex and building up general health, women can eventually live a bacterial vaginosis free life.

Conclusion

Other women and people in general can't understand what it is like to live with bacterial vaginosis, unless they have experienced it themselves. It can be a very isolating condition and it can come between partners in a relationship. One of the worst things can be the embarrassment of it all. This just adds to the isolation and can stop women seeking advice about their problem.

I hope that this book will have explained the situation for women as far as understanding bacterial vaginosis is concerned and how they can take back control of their lives. Once women know more about bacterial vaginosis the more that they can take control of its treatment. This can be from making sure that doctors and other medical staff take them seriously and do the right things to selecting home treatments and personal routines that prevent the condition coming back.

One important thing to remember is that there are lots of women out there that are suffering exactly the same thing and that by talking to other people with bacterial vaginosis we can also help ourselves. This talking and exchanging ideas could be in person, but more than likely, these days, might be within forums and specialized social network sites on the internet. In fact internet forums can be very good because they allow people to remain anonymous and in that way are more likely to talk about their problems, even if they are very embarrassing. These exchanges of ideas allow women to find out about new treatments and ideas that can be change makers for the future.

When looking at the vast array of treatments for bacterial vaginosis it is important to realize that not all treatments work for all women. This means that somebody who claims that a particular treatments work exceptionally well for them isn't being disingenuous. It is simply a case that everybody has a different reaction to both the infection and the treatment. For example a women with a mild case of bacterial vaginosis may be able to clear it up every time by just using probiotics. She will be very happy about this and will want to share her experience with other women in the hope that it will help them too. This same scenario may however, be very frustrating for a woman who finds that probiotics are absolutely no use to them at all. It is a case of matching the treatment to your own particular case.

Hopefully this book has given lots of ideas for women to try in their search for their perfect treatment. However, women should also keep an eye on those forums and news items for other treatments that may have been found. Keep up to date and you might find the ideal cure for you. Recently I even found a case where a woman had accidently found that her bacterial vaginosis could be dealt with using an hemorrhoid cream. This was only found out because she was using it for its real use at the time. On my part I can only wish you the success that you need in order to find your perfect cure. As for me, I swear by Apple Cider Vinegar for just about everything as people who have read my book on this topic will have seen.

About the Author

Ellen Vincent has written a number of other books. The first book complements this 'Bacterial Vaginosis' book because it gives more of the background as to why green smoothies are so healthy and how to make them. The second book details the health benefits of Apple cider vinegar. Both books are published as paperbacks and on the kindle platform.

Green smoothies are very popular when it comes to dieting, detoxifying and giving the human body the nutrients that it needs in order to work at the peak of performance. This book explains the many ways that green smoothies can help your body and improve your health and life in general. There are plenty of tips on producing and tailoring green smoothies for your individual needs and there are over 100 exciting recipe ideas included in the book.

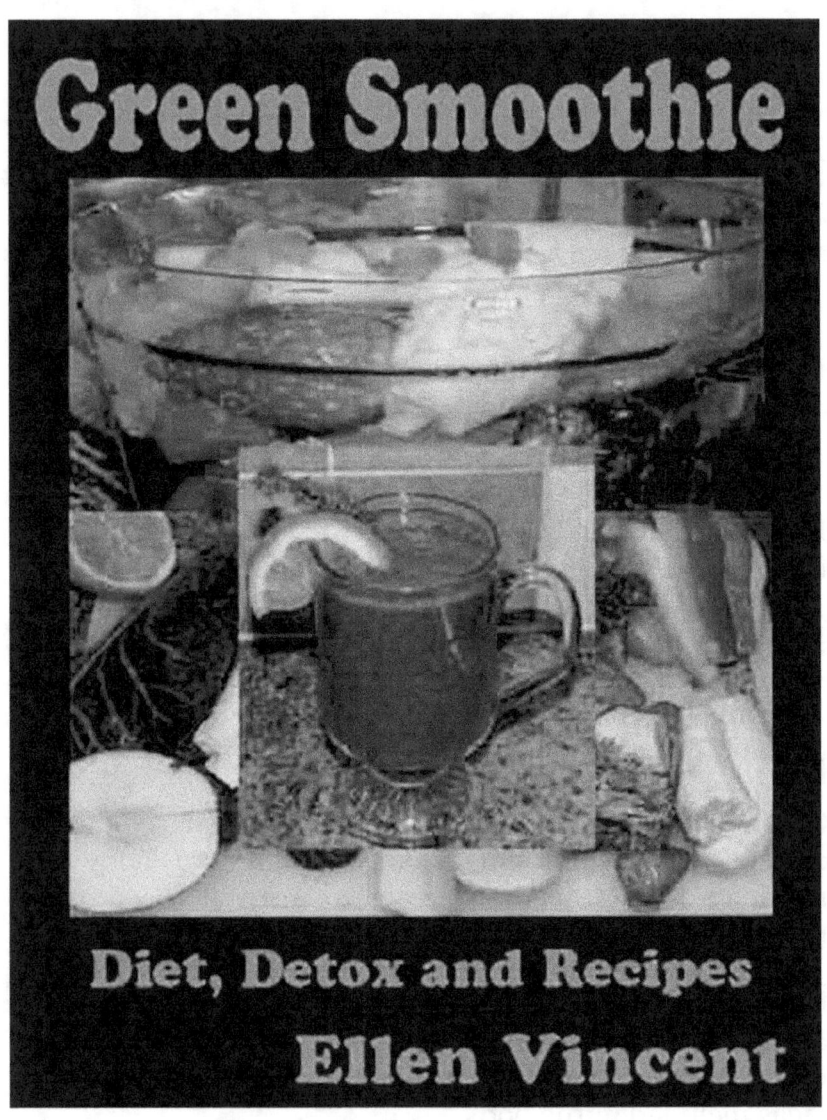

Green Smoothie

Diet, Detox and Recipes

Ellen Vincent

Green smoothies give you all of your nutrients the way that nature intended. This means that they are all in their raw form without chemicals, additives and processing. In basic terms you get more out your food when it is consumed in this way. This is because raw food contains more vital nutrients such as vitamins, antioxidants and amino acids. These are so good for your body that people who start eating them can experience a natural high as they are rapidly used up and turned into valuable materials. This means that green smoothies make you feel good as well as doing good.

Green smoothies are a valuable tool when it comes to dieting and losing weight. Due to the fact that they can make you feel fuller for longer they can help you to rapidly lose weight. They can also be the answer to the dieting plateau that many people reach on a normal low calorie diet. There are many other ways that green smoothies can enhance a diet or help in losing weight.

Green Smoothies could be your body's answer to those niggling health problems that can make life a misery. Modern life itself can have a bad effect on the human body and that includes the food that we eat. In seems that the further that we get away from nature, the more problems that we appear to have. If you look back to our ancestors they didn't have supermarkets and chemical additives to preserve and enhance the flavours and appearance of the foods they ate. You have to ask yourself how much damage all of these chemical additives cause? In addition to this even cooking foods causes chemical changes to happen to food and this can result in substances forming which can be bad for us and can even cause certain cancers.

If you feel like life is getting on top of you after too many 'little indulgencies' then green smoothies can be used as a way of detoxifying the body and rapidly returning it to normality.

Green Smoothie provides you with all of the information that you need to get your body working as nature intended. Get the book and join in this exciting new world of health.

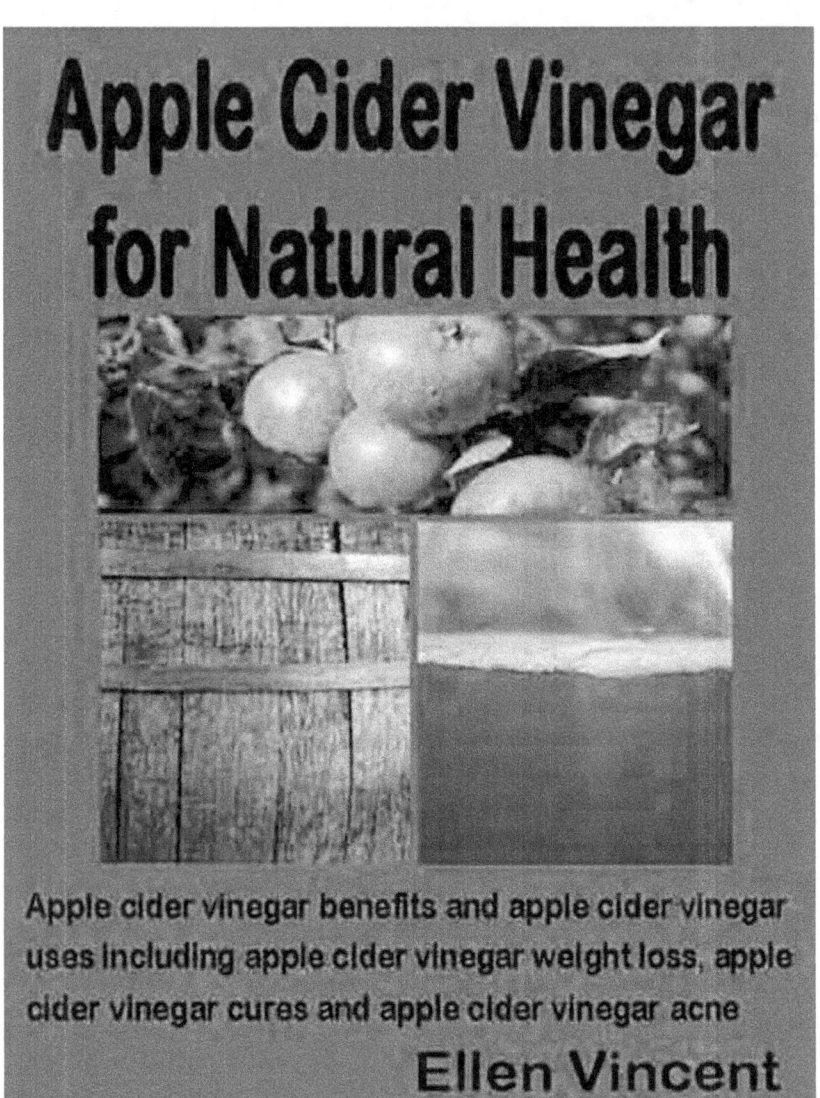

Apple Cider Vinegar for Natural Health

Apple cider vinegar benefits and apple cider vinegar uses including apple cider vinegar weight loss, apple cider vinegar cures and apple cider vinegar acne

Ellen Vincent

Apple cider vinegar for natural health is all about how you can use this wonderful natural health tonic to improve your life. Apple cider vinegar has been used for centuries to treat a whole host of illnesses and conditions. These cures and remedies have become part of our folklore, but that doesn't mean that we shouldn't take them seriously. Apple cider vinegar contains many health giving substances such as vitamins, minerals, antioxidants, bioflavenoids and of course the main ingredient of acetic acid. All of these things can help our bodies to work to the peak of performance and shrug off some of those day to day conditions that get us down. You can drink apple cider vinegar or apply it directly to the skin or hair. Either way you are getting the benefit of all of these super nutrients. Some books on apple cider vinegar are written by the people who are then trying to sell the vinegar to you. I am not involved in selling these products at all. My main interest comes from my scientific and educational background together with the fact that I use apple cider vinegar myself on many occasions during my day to day life. I am a real fan and take a daily tonic to ward off illness. I also use it on my skin and hair to great effect. I am so impressed with the results that I get with apple cider vinegar that I felt compelled to research it further and then write this book. I have never come across one single substance with so many uses before, and the results can often be stunning. So, take while and look at the information in the book and then try apple cider vinegar for yourself. Pretty soon you could become a real fan too!

This version 2 of the book contains extra information, and in particular details about how to use apple cider vinegar in your daily cooking. There are plenty of recipes and cookery ideas that you can try out for yourself.